SAG]

How To Be An Older Woman

Clare Shaw

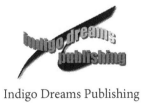

Indigo Dreams Publishing

First Edition: SAGEISM; How To Be An Older Woman
First published in Great Britain in 2015 by:
Indigo Dreams Publishing Ltd
24 Forest Houses
Halwill
Beaworthy
EX21 5UU
www.indigodreams.co.uk

ISBN 978-1-909357-70-9

The views expressed in this book do not necessarily reflect those of
the publishers.
This book is a work of fiction and, except in the case of historical
fact, any resemblance to actual persons, living or dead, is purely
coincidental.

Designed and typeset in Minion Pro by Indigo Dreams.
Cover design by Ronnie Goodyer at Indigo Dreams
Images from Dreamstime.com
Printed and bound in Great Britain by 4edge Ltd.
www.4edge.co.uk.
*Papers used by Indigo Dreams are recyclable products made from
wood grown in sustainable forests following the guidance of the Forest
Stewardship Council*

To my cousins Joss and Ros - two feisty and inspirational women in their prime.

ACKNOWLEDGEMENTS

Thank you to all the women and men in their middle years who talked to me about their concerns and achievements and inspired me to write this book.

CONTENTS

SAGEISM

How To Be An Older Woman

INTRODUCTION

Sageism is a celebration of growing older and wiser. It's a desire for a society that reveres the wisdom of experience and is an alternative to the current climate where middle-aged and older women are judged simply by whether they've managed to look ten years younger than they are. Not much of an achievement if it all came about by lucky genes or a surgeon with an eye on his or her bank balance. So let's celebrate getting older - after all, it's so much better than the alternative.

Women who have reached middle-age, and I'm one of them, are too often made to feel invisible and are consequently retreating into dark corners. It's about time we came out into the light and shouted about how great older women are and how much they have to contribute to this society, which is sadly still rife with ageism and sexism.

The time is right for this. There are many examples in this book of middle-aged women being discriminated against or ridiculed. But the tide is beginning to turn. Attitudes show some small signs of changing, and we must keep that momentum going. We need to learn how to live our lives as middle-aged women with confidence in a world that mostly wants equality even if it's going the long way round to get there. The trouble with tides turning is we can miss it and get stranded, or we can get swept along with a feeling of being out of control. So let's ride the waves and create a few of our own. Last cliché. Promise. Well almost.

It should be easy to be an older woman. There is, after all, some truth in the maxims – 'older and wiser' and we 'mellow with age'. We've been around a few decades and we may not have seen it all but we've seen a fair sized chunk of it. We must have learnt something from our mistakes and we're, well, calmer somehow. More measured, less frenzied. Unless we're having a bit of a hormone imbalance episode of course. (See, we can even

11

poke fun at ourselves.)

Why does it feel like we've got the double-barrelled shotgun of ageism and sexism pointing straight at us, making us eager to hide away and keep out of the firing line? When we should be catching the bullets in our teeth, spitting them out and saying – yes, I'm older, yes I'm a woman. AND I'M GLAD. But we don't say that we're pleased to be an older woman. All right, we might whisper it but there's usually a loud voice inside our heads drowning it out by shouting that it would be better if we were younger. Just a tad. Well a few years, really. In fact knock a couple of decades off and we'll all be happy. Why? Where is the logic in being ashamed of being older? Why do so many of us suffer from failed-to-be-young syndrome?

It's like being ashamed of having two feet or being embarrassed that Wednesday follows Tuesday. How can we be ashamed of not inventing a clock that ticks slowly back in time until we eventually crawl back into our mother's womb? We might as well be ashamed we didn't quite manage to connect with alien life forms and create a new species. WE'RE BEING ASHAMED, EMBARRASSED AND IN DENIAL OF THE MOST NATURAL THING IN THE WORLD. Yes, we all get older.

This is a book which will celebrate being a middle-aged and older woman, while acknowledging that we exist in a society which seems intent on doing the opposite. We have been excluded from so many aspects of society, from modelling clothes to presenting on television, from being listened to as an expert in our field to performing on stage. The old song tells us to 'keep young and beautiful if you want to be loved.' Why? Isn't it about time we challenged both the obvious and the subtle ageism and sexism in our society so we can regain our rightful place in the world and hold our heads up with real confidence. It's no good sitting at home whinging about it all, we all have to play our part in ensuring attitudes are changed so we must all GET OUT

THERE AND LIVE. Live our lives the way we want to and not how we are told we ought to. And if all this sounds a bit earnest, then fear not because we are going to have a laugh together as we take this journey. Did I just write 'journey'? Sorry, I won't write it again. Or inner child. It's really not that sort of book.

ONE: TOWARDS DEATH

Most of you will be put off by the chapter title. You may even be tempted to skip the chapter completely. DON'T. I'm not suggesting that being middle-aged means you have to start measuring yourself up for a coffin and write instructions to your children to make sure Auntie Susan doesn't get the oak chest. I mean that the D word, which is avoided by everyone of all ages, needs to be addressed. It's part of the problem.

Let's go back to the introduction. No need to flick back a page. I'll repeat it here and add three little words onto the end. So here it is – we're ashamed, embarrassed and in denial of the most natural thing in the world. Yes, we all get older and THEN WE DIE. So, not as good as 'I love you' for three little words but much more likely to be honest and not likely to ever change. Presumably, no one wants to miss out the getting older part of that sequence. So there you have it. We are all on the way to death and getting older is part of that. We can't change it, all we can do is embrace it.

To be clear, I know there are occasions when people die young and that is the saddest of all events. Obviously it is. Because just like we always say when it happens – they died too soon, before their time. It was the wrong order of things. So what's the alternative to an undeniably tragic early death? It's to GROW OLD FIRST.

There, that wasn't difficult, was it? We've managed to talk about death – one of the greatest taboos in our western culture. Particularly in Britain. We've even used the proper word for it – death. Not 'gone to a better place' or 'passed on' or the potentially confusing, 'gone away'. And definitely not 'gone into the fertiliser business' or 'taken the escalator to a different floor'. Just death. There are hundreds of euphemisms, many of which seem to deny death completely – 'fallen asleep' is seen engraved on a multitude of gravestones as if, any minute, a corpse will wake up and wonder which practical joker has shovelled a load of dirt on top of her. The ultimate denial is spending your life savings on having your head frozen so you can be revived just as soon as we've found that cure for cancer, Alzheimer's or, well, death. This is the modern day equivalent of the Egyptians leaving food in the pyramids in case their dead kings get a bit peckish in the night.

Interestingly, cultures which embrace death and spend a long time with the dead and dying – from the funeral pyres in Asia, to Buddhists spending days or weeks helping the soul find a good new life – tend to embrace old age as well. It isn't only ancient tribes who value the experience of old age and revere their ageing population – Buddhists, Jews and many Asian cultures do it too. The word for an older person in Japan is Oji San which translates as venerable one. That's way better than batty old granny.

Perhaps if we are going to start respecting people as they get older, we need to start embracing death. This means accepting that it will happen, talking about it and making it part of our culture. Instead of pretending that it's something that happens to other people. We can't all be Peter Pan. Cliff Richard's got the monopoly on that.

Apparently more than two thirds of us never make any plans for what happens to us after we die. We really should get round to sitting down over a cup of tea and talking about what we want. But it seems the British aren't very good at that. Talking about death, I mean. We're expert on the sitting down with a cup of tea part. I suppose the weather outside the window just seems a more important topic somehow.

There are signs, however, that we are beginning to embrace death and it's started in, of all places, America. Yes, the land where cars toot their horns behind funeral corteges to get them to drive faster. The death café, which started in the States, has now come to England and while there are, at the time of writing, only a handful of such events, perhaps it might represent a slight change in attitude towards death and the dying. No longer something to speak of in hushed tones, whispering 'I'm so sorry for your loss' as if using a code for a drugs deal, death is finally something to talk about over a brew and a Battenburg. And I decided to give it a try.

Before continuing along these lines, I sense some of you may be wondering why I am confusing middle-aged with the dying. We can't all have blocked arteries. As I explained, the cultures who embrace death respect their elderly. And if they respect their elderly, they respect the experience of each and every individual. The number of years we have been alive matters BECAUSE IT MEANS WE HAVE EXPERIENCE TO SHARE. And if you respect the older generation, chances are you respect the disabled, the mentally ill, children, babies, the lot. So, maybe, instead of saying – it's a youth culture but let's see if we can at least extend that acceptance to people in their thirties or, at a push, forties, we start with death and move backwards. If we can revere a ninety year old on her death bed, valuing the contributions of the middle-aged is going to be a doddle.

So, back to the death café where an Earl Grey awaits me. The tea, not the dead 19th century Prime Minister, although that might have given a new meaning to the death café movement. I felt rather nervous as I walked towards the chosen location for the event. I'm not sure why, perhaps because death café sounds like a film where an innocent bystander takes shelter from the pouring rain in a quiet, out of the way café only to be confronted with the sound of cellos, indicating that at least one person is destined to die. Just as that thought arrived in my mind, it started pouring with rain and I was feeling decidedly like that innocent bystander. I gulped, opened the door and was greeted by the sound of laughter. I immediately realised that I hadn't been expecting laughter, wailing maybe but not laughter. But then that's how deep our fear of death goes. It's always been something to talk about in hushed tones, presumably because if the dead heard us, they'd leap out from under the table, saying 'No, it's not like that at all.'

There was a welcoming array of cakes on the table and steaming pots of tea and coffee. Bright coloured napkins and a vase of sunflowers adorned the table, perhaps to distinguish it from a funeral spread. A young man of around thirty called Jason welcomed me and urged me to 'tuck in before it's too late.' Did he know something I didn't? Then I realised he meant tuck in before everyone else ate the cakes. Two women were discussing their recipes for carrot cake and a young couple were talking about the first time they'd ever made brownies together. I couldn't help wondering if I'd inadvertently come to a branch meeting of the Great British Bake Off. What had all this to do with death? Unless Jason was trying to up our cholesterol intake so one of us might experience it and report back to the others.

'Hi, I'm Clare,' I said to the young couple, who introduced themselves as Josie and Michael, 'is this your first time?' Well, it sounded like the right thing to say. Josie told me it was their second meeting and that they had actually met at the last meeting and were now a couple. Something to tell their children, I suppose – Mummy and Daddy met at a death event where we realised we shared the same sense of humour.

'Did you come in order to meet someone, then?' I asked, wondering what sort of partner you were looking for if you went to a death café to find him or her. I was quite relieved when they said no. But when Michael then explained that he'd always been fascinated by death, I felt slightly uncomfortable. Those pre-conceived ideas coming through, I suppose.

Then something struck me. Michael and Josie were

talking to me as if I WAS A NORMAL PERSON. Which I obviously am, but what I mean was that they seemed unaware and unfazed that I was a middle-aged woman. I DIDN'T FEEL INVISIBLE AT ALL. Maybe my theory was correct – accept your own death and you will start to respect those nearer to it than you.

Jason tapped the edge of the cup with a teaspoon and coughed. The group fell silent and Michael reached for Josie's hand. I just stopped myself in time from also reaching for Josie's hand as if trying to contact the dead. But that wasn't on the agenda at all and instead, Jason began to read the minutes of the last death meeting. They had apparently debated reincarnation, praised the hospice movement, discussed Dignitas, elected a death secretary, wondered how they could get more members to attend and ate cake. All this and Michael and Josie still had time to assess each other's coffin size.

I looked around the group. Apart from our young-couple-in-love and Jason, there was an elderly woman who nodded so vigorously at everything Jason said, I thought her head might roll under the table. Later, I found out she was his mother and started to imagine that conversation where Jason jollily invited her to a death café. And as for the Dignitas discussion – it doesn't bear thinking about. And there I am with my prejudices again, assuming an older person doesn't want to talk about death in case everyone thinks it's about her. A woman of about forty with orange hair wearing a large sack, a nervous looking thin man of about thirty with thick, black ringed glasses and a bubbly woman of a similar age with curly hair and a polka dot dress made up the rest of the group.

During the evening, I managed to ask each of them why they had come and the main reason seemed to be a fascination with death. They were in the right place then. The man in the black rimmed glasses turned out to be a Buddhist so that made sense. Polka dot dress also went to séances and Jason himself had done a PHD in death. An expert in dying then. He should make short shrift of it when his time came. It was a smaller group than expected but a lively one. I can quite honestly say, I have never laughed so much in my life. We discussed death rituals from different countries which Jason was something of an expert on and we discussed what songs we would like at our funerals. After a serious discussion, Another One Bites the Dust and Knock on Wood were suggested, along with Living In A Box and 50 Ways To Leave Your Lover. I'm On Fire was put forward as a choice for cremations. As I said, there was a lot of laughter.

Perhaps that's the secret - laugh at what you fear. And I shall return to that theme because it isn't only death we can laugh at (not actually at the funeral or anything). We can also laugh at ourselves getting older. We had a wonderful evening with some interesting discussions where I learnt so much. At the time, I hardly noticed that we spanned the decades between us. We were drawn together by a common interest and I imagined that other groups drawn together by something in common could also put age to one side. I am now aware that this isn't always the case. Still, at least I know it can be done.

And so to Richard the third. Yes, the one who turned up in the car park in Leicester without so much as a ticket. Largely thanks to Shakespeare, he has always been thought of as a bad king. With some evidence of course. He was a murderer by all accounts and so the label seems appropriate. But when his bones were dug up, great excitement swept the country and he became something of a minor celebrity. I half expected his bones to turn up as a guest on Loose Women. Soon after, there followed revelations that he may have been misunderstood and he was quite nice really. Just an ordinary hunchback and the victim of a bad assessment by ATOS who declared he was fit to go into battle at Bosworth. And the matter of those little murders had been greatly exaggerated, so much so that he may have been one of our greatest monarchs.

That's what happens. Someone dies and they become a saint. I remember when my father died, my mother declared that she could not go on without him as their marriage had been a perfect example of romantic bliss. And true to her promise, she died about nine weeks later. Clearly, everyone who knew her told me, she had died of a broken heart. I even found myself believing it until I remembered all the crockery that had flown past their ears, all the harsh words that had been screamed at each other and my mother's refusal to celebrate their golden wedding anniversary on the grounds that she had had a miserable life. It didn't seem like the recipe for dying of a broken heart, not to mention the fact that her liver had packed up due to the large amount of sherry she had been consuming on a daily basis for the previous forty years. Dying of a broken liver doesn't quite have the same ring to it. In the weeks following their deaths, everyone told me how perfect they both were. Not that I wanted people to say, 'I really liked your father but he had a terrible temper' or 'your mother was a good friend but rather judgemental.' But it wasn't just that we were wanting to remember their good points, we genuinely forgot their faults and they became saintly and angelic overnight. I found myself telling a complete stranger the other day how close I was to my parents. I wasn't. I miss them and love them but we really weren't close and they really weren't perfect. I have just paused over the delete button writing this. I feel terrible admitting to the world that my parents had faults. Why? EVERYONE HAS FAULTS. The problem is, we don't like to speak ill of the dead.

Hang on, why is that a problem? Isn't that what we should do with the living as well? Focus on their good points, accept their faults and see the angel inside everyone? I think of my parents in a far more positive way than when they were alive.

And I even feel some affection for Richard the third. I felt quite moved at Thatcher's funeral even though I hated all her policies and everything she stood for. Why? Why this apparent change of mind when someone dies? I don't think it is a change of mind, it's a shift of viewpoint. Once people are gone, we can look at someone's life like a story. We can see the person's motivations – why they did what they did, and we can say well done, you got to the end of the race.

My daughter, Emma, runs and has occasionally taken part in a marathon. She doesn't expect to win or anything but she does the best she can, gets fit and faster and has fun. When she gets to the finishing line, my husband and I are cheering very loudly and, embarrassingly, we cry with pride, shouting out to complete strangers – that's our daughter and she's run a marathon. Then we cheer everyone else who gets to the end. Whether they're first or three hundred and first, we cheer. Because they made it. Emma sometimes says she made a mistake and set off too quickly or forgot to take enough energy gels on board but SO WHAT? She still got to the end. Sometimes, we meet people who have had to pull out of the race early because they hadn't trained properly or had an injury. We still pat them on the back and say well done. Because they took part and did their best most of the time. Like life. You can only do your best most of the time. And when it's over, everyone deserves a pat on the back. With the exception of Hitler and people of his ilk, I suppose.

With a few notable exceptions, we congratulate the dead. We can still acknowledge their faults but with compassion and humour. One of my mother's faults was making us eat an appalling trifle at every family get together. So my sister-in-law made a similar one for her funeral and we all laughed at her cooking (my mother's not my sister-in-law's). But with, I hope, a great deal of affection. My father had a temper and all credit to him, it improved as he mellowed with age. He ended up as very gentle and thoughtful. I love thinking of him in his later years. And as for the temper, I was able to laugh with my brothers at his habit of trying to hit us in the back of the car while driving. As I was in the middle, I invariably got the worst of it which was grossly unfair as it was inevitably one of my brothers who had said or done something that warranted the punishment. My father, however, would be satisfied he had found a target and carry on driving. And yes, I can remember this with affection. I can even say it helped me go out of my way to be fair to my daughters and to try and deal with problems calmly. (Note to daughters, I said try, I didn't say I always succeeded.)

We have it in us to accept people and look on their faults with affection and even love. It's just that we tend to wait until they're dead to do it. Of course, once someone is dead, it is easier to accept because it's too late to change anything. But we can start accepting people's foibles while they're still alive. There may be times when we want to help someone to change a fault. BUT WE CAN STILL START FROM THE POINT OF COMPASSION AND UNDERSTANDING.

How does this fit in with the middle-aged who have not yet booked their trip to the big reality show in the sky? Oops, and there was me arguing against euphemisms. All right, how does this fit in with me and my peers? The not nearly ready to die. I feel a list coming on.

1. Laugh at your own faults and people will laugh along with you.
2. Remember that life is like a Marathon – taking part will get you the congratulations you deserve. Eventually.
3. You are probably three quarters of the way through the Marathon. Of course you feel tired and wonder if it's worth it. It is. And look how far you've come.

4. Think of someone you knew who is now dead. Now think of yourself with that same measured affection and acceptance.
5. And think of others that way too.
6. Go to a death café and encourage others to do the same.
7. Remind yourself you're going to die (but maybe not just before you go to sleep at night.)
8. Live each day as if it's your last but keep stocked up on milk and bread, just in case.
9. Talk about death to people as you chat over the water dispenser at work or as you make conversation after your yoga class. Talk about it naturally as you would any other topic. Do your small bit towards making it normal to discuss it.
10. Remember that death is always looming.

Ah, I feel some explanation of the last point is called for. We are all going to die. You may feel that you are nearer to death than you were ten years ago and of course, you are. But the truth is, death can come and tap on your shoulder at any time – we don't have a sell by date stamped on the back of our necks. You could make a guess about when you are going to die. Say, you've always been in good health and both your parents have lived to a ripe old age, then it might be reasonable to assume you could reach your nineties. BUT YOU MIGHT NOT. So, don't waste your time, enjoy every minute. I know that sounds obvious, but let's look at the lessons given to us by those who know they have limited life.

There have been numerous books written in recent years where authors have gathered the regrets of the dying and interviewed people who know they have limited time left in this world. Suffice to say, the dying quickly learn to appreciate every single moment of their life. They notice every flower, every insect and despite the weeks running out, take time to look at these things and take in every detail. Given a death sentence, they become mindful and live every day as if it is their last, because, frankly, it might be. The dying all report that so long as the pain can be controlled, they really were enjoying each moment. SO WHY NOT LIVE LIKE THAT NOW? After all, we're all on our way to death. We don't know when or how in most cases, but we are dying. We all have limited time. The oldest person ever lived for 122 years, so it's unlikely you'll live beyond that. So there you are, however optimist you are, there are limits.

Children cannot wait to reach their next birthday, often proudly adding three quarters to their age in their bid to press on in life. This changes sometime in our twenties when suddenly we want time to stand still. In our middle years, we definitely don't want to get older too quickly. I think this can be looked on as a positive thing. We can't slow time up but we can make it seem as if it's slowed up. How? Let's switch briefly from the lessons of the dying to the lessons of children.

When we are young, time seems to go slower and then speeds up so every year appears to rush past more quickly. This is because life for a child is full of new experiences. Pretty well everything they do is novel for them. But as we get older, our lives become repetitions of familiar routines. Have you noticed how when you go on holiday the week seems longer than the previous one you spent at work? This is because you've had a week of new places, people and experiences. Like a child does all the time. I am not suggesting you need to jack in your job, take out a huge bank loan and go round the world (though, why not?). But learn from the dying woman who looks in detail at every flower and insect because like a child, she is also finding new experiences. She is noticing things she has never noticed before. She is creating new experiences without leaving her home and garden. So start slowing up your world simply by being mindful.

The other lesson from the dying is looking at their

regrets. Again these have been well documented in books on the subject. But let me list some of the things the dying didn't wish they'd done. None of them wished they had:

Worked harder.
Whinged more about being old/middle-aged.
Rushed about more.
Pretended there was no such thing as death.
Lied about their age.
Used Botox/ had cosmetic surgery.
Hidden themselves away.
Apologised for themselves more.
Kept their kitchen cupboards tidier.
Cleaned the car more often.

So, time for a more positive list.

1. Remember you are dying. You could die next week (we can say that now we're good at talking about death.) So live each moment and seize the day.
2. Study mindfulness. Do activities which encourage mindfulness such as yoga and meditation. A fuller life does not have to involve cramming more stuff in.
3. Spend time with people older than you. You can learn from them in the same way as you have experience to pass down to the generation below.
4. Write your own obituary. What do you want people to remember you for? So be that person and do whatever you need to do (I doubt you want to be remembered for working too hard or having a neat kitchen).
5. Plan your funeral. I bet you want people to celebrate your life. Doing this will help you look back and celebrate your achievements so far.

It may seem strange to start a book about being middle-aged/older/in that awkward section of life between adolescence and memory loss, by looking at death. But if we know where we're heading, it can help us make sense of where we are. If we want to pass our experience down to the next generation, then we have to find out what we can learn from the dead and dying. If you're climbing a mountain, you will see yourself in relation to the peak. Maybe you had to change path on route, maybe you needed to slow down as you approached half-way, maybe you wanted to stop and take in the view, but you will always think in terms of how far from the peak you are.

You may be half way there, three quarters of the way or maybe you have the end in sight. So accept that. You wouldn't pretend you were near the bottom of that mountain if you were on a climbing expedition.

At the time of writing I am fifty six. As I'm unlikely to live till one hundred and twelve, I am more than half way through the expected number of years. I am over half way towards that mountain peak. I have had cancer twice and a pulmonary embolism so I am aware that anything could happen to bring death nearer. It nearly has. I will do what it takes to stop that happening but at the same time, I will not put things off that I want to do. Just in case. I have fifty six years of experience behind me. I am proud of some of the things I've done, not so proud of others. But overall, it's been a great journey so far and I am looking forward to the rest.

And surprise, surprise, I look fifty six. Not forty six and not sixty six but fifty six. I remember things from the sixties that other people can't. There are things I can't do now that I could do when I was younger (pretend to be under 16 to get a cheaper ticket, French skipping, remember where I left the remote control, dance to Billie Jean, do a passable impression of Dusty Springfield) but equally, there are plenty of things I can do now which I couldn't when I was younger (pretend to be sixty to get a cheaper ticket, use a computer, celebrate my thirtieth wedding anniversary, say venerable one in Japanese, relate the plots of every Haruki Murakami novel, sing in tune.) Actually, I still can't sing in tune but it sounds in tune since my hearing isn't as good as it used to be.

Why would I pretend to be younger and deny the journey I've made so far? Why pretend to be less experienced? Somewhere along the way, getting older has become something to be sad and regretful about. Part of that is that we don't want to die made worse by the fact that we never acknowledge death happens to us all. So accept death, live your life knowing it's going to happen and live as if it might be just round the corner. Also, learn from the dying and the way we revere the already dead. Happy to be middle-aged/older now? I thought not. Just as well, really, or this book would end at chapter one and wouldn't be a book at all. Just a pamphlet. About death. Might as well be a leaflet from some obscure religion which I would have to deliver door to door.

So, on we go with our manual for the middle-aged woman. And while I've got my mother in my mind, let's think about how being older has changed since the last generation.

TWO: WHAT WE LEARNT FROM OUR MOTHERS

Everything's changed since our mothers' day. Being middle-aged certainly has. In fact even the time you hit middle-age has changed. Life expectancy goes up with each generation, so that we can expect to live at least eight more years than our mothers used to. Men's life expectancy has gone up even more – by ten years in the last fifty years – as they slowly catch us up. On average, we can expect to live until 89 and our male partners until 85. And so many people are reaching their hundredth birthday, ten new candle factories have opened up, and the Queen has repetitive strain injury from signing all those cards. So it stands to reason that if death has been pushed on, then the middle of our life must be later too.

In fact we know this just by looking at pictures of our mothers. By forty, they were dressed in a kind of grey and beige uniform, with permed hair to match. They sported teeth, glasses and floral aprons, all of which were removed for an afternoon nap. Now we raid our daughter's wardrobes, have no idea what the natural colour of our hair is and only have a nap in the afternoon because we've had a late night out, clubbing maybe. We laugh at pictures of our frumpy mothers and assume (probably wrongly) that our daughters will look at us in years to come and see a youthful, trendy icon of fashion and coolness.

We are actually quite muddled as to when being middle-aged starts and ends. It's a very grey area, but no longer literally. That's because our mothers' generation tended to do things in the same order and at the same time. In the fifties and early sixties, women mostly saw marriage as the only option and career women were still a little confused about whether they could mix this in with a successful marriage. Most women got married in their twenties. The average age to marry in the 1950s was 22. These days, the range of when you get married or become a couple is more varied, mostly later than in days gone by and often just in time to stop the biological clock running out. The average age for getting married is now 30. But 20 or 40 or even later will do very nicely too, thank you.

We are having babies later too. In the 1950s the average age for having a baby was 22, whereas it's 30 today. Again, there is a bigger age range today for having children. I recall a girl in my class at school having a mother who looked like my grandmother. She was called Angela and had two grown up sisters. My own mother explained that Angela was probably a mistake. As she farted rather a lot in PE lessons, I was rather inclined to agree with her. Angela's mother seemed rather embarrassed about the situation and used to stand at the school gate, hiding her face behind her string shopping bag. These days anything goes and with more second families arriving as part of a new relationship, older mothers (and fathers) are commonplace and no one cares or judges (mostly).

Life is changing as well, and always will. It is impossible to compare ourselves to our own mothers when we have more choices. In the nineteen fifties and sixties, women tended to think they had a choice between motherhood and a career. It was beginning to change, but more mothers gave up work while they had pre-school children. And with the pill not being available to all until 1961, there were often a lot of pre-school children in a family (see Call the Midwife). Men are more hands on as fathers now and often share the childcare or are house husbands. There are so many more different types of families now with step children, step parents, same sex parents, stay at home fathers as well as an increasing number of women and men choosing to live the single life – a third of us, in fact. Anything goes and with variation comes less judgement, I like to think. So middle-aged starts, well, anytime you want really.

With our lives being so very different, is there really

anything we can learn from our mothers? We can learn from their mistakes for a start. As I've explained, there is no clear age any more for when middle-age kicks in. There probably never was but in our mothers' time, they insisted that at 40, everything had to change. I remember my own mother crying her eyes out when she hit the big Four-O. It seemed more of a milestone then than it does now. These days it's an excuse for a party, back then it was an excuse to buy more grey cardigans, put your hair in a neat, grey bun and complain about creaky bones, piles and young-people-today. So:-

Lesson number one: MIDDLE-AGE IS FLEXIBLE. It no longer has to be at 40, it no longer has to be any particular time. AND NOTHING NEEDS TO CHANGE. Unless we want it to, of course.

Lesson number two: ANYTHING GOES. We now have fewer pre-conceived ideas about being middle-aged or older. You don't have to change the way you dress, behave or live your life as you get older. BUT YOU CAN IF YOU WANT. If you want to go clubbing at fifty, then go. If you want to make jam then make jam. Wear what you want, work as long as you want, and take part in any activity that takes your fancy from sewing to skateboarding, from pottery to naked parachute jumping.

Lesson number three: NOTHING STAYS THE SAME. Life is changing faster now that at any time in our history. Our mothers had to spend longer on housework because they were probably pre-dishwasher, pre-microwave and pre-let's spray the house with Febreze and no one will notice the dust. They didn't have access to the information we do via the Internet, where we can view middle-aged celebrities who have set a trend for not looking or behaving middle-aged (a double edged sword which we will talk about later.) We are not like our mothers because our lives and the world around us ARE COMPLETELY DIFFERENT. So be different and don't model yourself on your mother at your age (even though she stares back at you every time you look in the mirror).

Lesson number four: All your mothers will be a little different. OK, so they are more likely to have married younger, had children younger and let themselves be the epitome of middle-agedness by about forty. But even if you can recognise your mother from this average, and I can, each one will be different. I bet your mother didn't drink as much sherry as mine, for example. So think about your own mother and think of the ways YOU DO NOT WANT TO BE LIKE HER. So, I don't drink sherry, I am more broad minded, less judgemental, more willing to try new experiences and will never ever have a perm that makes me look like petrified poodle with its paw in the electric socket. You will learn your own individual don'ts from your own mother.

Lesson number five: DON'T LET YOUTH CULTURE TAKE THE STEERING WHEEL. Let's look at this in detail.

I really don't know which generation is to blame for this but at some point the older generation who made the decisions and dictated what happened in society, gave way to the young. Presumably it was when the youth started having their own disposable income. In the 1900s, there was no such thing as a teenager – just children and adults. Then during the 1930s and 40s, staying longer in education meant young people began to see themselves as a group with their own particular needs and viewpoints.

Arguably the teenager was invented in the post war years of the 1950s as a previously untapped market of new consumers. And with teenage years also associated with breaking free of the older generation, youth fashion and style became paramount to their identity. The 60s also saw youth challenging the status quo, looking for peace and understanding and demonstrating against anything that did not meet their ideals. Somewhere along the way, the young were the ones to be revered and the next generation up were accused of being out of touch. We became separated and people were categorised and judged by their age.

Take Valerie Singleton. Remember her? When I was growing up, she was one of the presenters on Blue Peter, along with Christopher Trace who no one remembers (probably not even Valerie Singleton). I think John Noakes was in there somewhere too, inventing the catch phrase 'Get down Shep.' This was not his pet name for Valerie but an instruction to his over excited Border Collie to stop him trying to roger Valerie's leg. Anyway, it's Valerie who all of us of a certain generation remember. She had a real authority about her, like one of those teachers you can't help admiring even though they have the bossiness gene, popular among our educators. If Val told you to collect milk bottle tops, you stole them off other people's doorsteps to get enough. If she showed you how to make a Christmas table decoration out of loo rolls, sticky back plastic and pictures cut out of your mother's catalogue, you assumed that, like homework, this was obligatory. Val was 35 when she joined Blue Peter and 45 when she left. Young, but a lot older than the viewers and she was WHAT WE EXPECTED. She was not particularly trendy and seemed to get on better with Princess Anne (not the epitome of fashion or new ideas) than any pop star who might be on the programme. She was, however, a very good and professional presenter. Leap ahead to today and a more recent presenter, Helen Skelton, started at age 25, ten years younger than Valerie Singleton. Also a good presenter, she talks, looks and oozes youth in the way Val never did. But she is WHAT WE EXPECT. We expect young presenters and young politicians and young, well everything. More about the age of women on TV later, but it seems worth looking at what our mothers watched on television and what we see. It's changed. And we need to keep our eye on that ball. Older women definitely need to claim back the areas of life which have become youth dominant since our mothers' day.

The things I like then about my own mother when she was middle-aged are:

1. She was less obsessed with trying to look younger. She definitely accepted the physical signs of getting older.
2. She expected to see older people in positions of power and influence (though most of them would have been male). Not only that, but what she thought of as young, we now regard as older. (See Valerie Singleton).
3. She seemed comfortable with her position in the family and society.

The things I don't like about my mother when she was middle-aged are:

1. She seemed to think there were rules about what a middle-aged woman should look like and how she behaved. Maybe there were – printed in the back of Good Housekeeping or Family Circle.
2. She thought men and women had clearly defined roles.
3. She thought it normal to slow down in middle-age. She saw middle-agedness as a limitation.
4. She liked to blend into the background.
5. She liked to say 'she's no better than she ought to be' and 'mutton dressed as lamb' in response to any of her contemporaries who threw away their grey cardigans and dyed their hair.
6. She was in awe of men in authority from the bank manager to the dentist.
7. She wore the same style of clothes and hair for decades. Perhaps she modelled herself on the Queen. She didn't get in

touch with her inner eccentric until it was nearly too late.

On balance, I think it might be better to be middle-aged now. But that doesn't mean we are not a section of society being at best sidelined and in many instances discriminated against.

What I don't know, of course, is what my mother thought about being middle-aged. I remember her crying on her fortieth birthday so she clearly didn't welcome it. However, she seemed to accept it and there were no signs that she fought against it. She did fight against her weight gain by wearing a girdle and eating strange diet rolls which were very light bread rolls with nothing in the middle. But she seemed to get frumpier on purpose (although interestingly she became more clothes conscious later in life). She did work but would never have allowed herself to be anything other than an additional income to my father's main income. She remained in a largely unhappy marriage as part of this general acceptance and she saw her main role as getting the dinner on the table for my father. She did not engage in feminism and I never really knew her views on the subject. Did she, like I sometimes do, feel invisible, pushed to the sidelines in this society? Did she feel discriminated against? Did she ever challenge the roles my father and her took on, based largely on their gender? I suspect not. I think ageism and sexism largely passed her by. As she died two years prior to writing this, it's too late to ask her and I need to know how typical she was. So off to see Brenda, now 80, just a couple of years younger than my mother would have been. Brenda was forty in 1970. Feminism was high on the agenda then, so did this affect Brenda's life, or did it bypass her completely as it had my mother?

So another trip to a café (not the death café this time, what with Brenda being eighty and having had some heart problems recently.) This time to meet an older woman who might be able to give me some insight as I help her to look back on her life.

I had already met Brenda, the mother of a friend of mine, a couple of times so I was aware that she likes a chat. Her mind is more alert than mine, as is her memory but I remembered that she struggled to walk a bit. She still drives although her daughter is contemplating confiscating her car. She's alert, and with glasses can see to drive all right but she's never got used to the amount of traffic in our town. Consequently she drives very slowly. And when reminded to use her indicators, explains that she knows which way she's going, thank you very much. So she was keen to meet in town and with her disabled badge was able to park outside the café I'd chosen. As it happens, she was more mobile than I'd remembered and practically ran in, waving her stick in the air and shouting, 'here I am, I've arrived.'

She had a strange felt hat on at a jaunty angle and wore a large coat despite it being the middle of summer. She had a shopping bag on wheels which she rammed into every table she passed, laughing like a drain every time she did so. It was then that I noticed two things about this eighty year old. Firstly, there was no way she wanted to fade into the background like I so often do and have done since hitting my fifties. And THE STAFF AND CUSTOMERS ALL SEEMED TO LOVE HER.

I looked around the café and noticed she had bought a smile to everyone's face. Meanwhile, the staff were rallying round her as if she was a VIP. I half expected them to sing God Save the Queen, curtsy and take some photos of themselves with Brenda to upload onto Facebook. So instead of the rather bland – 'here's a picture of me and you can just make out Simon Cowell in the background', they would be able to brag – 'here's me with an eccentric old woman called Brenda.'

Before we'd even started our in depth chat about middleageddom, I had learnt something already. YOU ARE

TREATED BETTER WHEN YOU ARE OLD THAN WHEN YOU ARE MIDDLE-AGED. There are limitations on that, of course - you have to be old and mostly independent. The newspapers are full of stories of abuse of the elderly. And once you are a vulnerable or sick elderly woman, then to be frank the chances that you won't always be treated well increase. But old women like Brenda, a little bit eccentric, clearly deaf and clumsy, needing a little bit of help but not too much and funny, well she was the bees knees as far as the café cliental and staff were concerned. I had arrived about ten minutes before her, skulked into a corner unnoticed and no one had come to take my order. They probably hadn't even realised I was there. Now there were waiting staff around us like the Paparazzi around a Middleton. Not surprising when I saw Brenda responding to them – she was, well, cute. But in a way a young child might be. And just because people were taking notice of her, DIDN'T MEAN SHE HAD A VOICE. Or that she is represented in business, politics and the media any more than the middle-aged are. And how long before Brenda turns from amusing to a burden?

How we treat our elderly once they need care is another book and we won't come out of it well in this society. Meanwhile, back to the middle-aged woman who is not in need of care, the woman like myself who can stand up for herself, who has the ability to be heard if only someone would listen. What does Brenda think of it all?

Coffees and cakes ordered, presented with care and good service to Brenda and practically thrown across the table at me, I start by asking Brenda if she remembers being in her forties and fifties. Luckily for this chapter, she does. She recalls that she was married to Geoff, who died four years ago and that she looked after him and their two children while also working part time in the library which she loved. She had trained as a librarian, ran the children's section of the library and had taken great pride in encouraging parents from all walks of life to come in and listen to stories and join a reading club she'd set up. It transpired that Brenda had turned down a promotion as she didn't want to increase her hours or take on more responsibility because she enjoyed being there for her children when they came home from school. At first the feminist in me had thoughts of inequality, suppression, and I-suppose-Geoff-was-in-the-pub. But Brenda had been given a choice and had confidently chosen the one that worked for her family. Nothing wrong with that.

Even so, I did ask if Geoff had done his share of looking after the kids.

'He worked long hours so I did most of it, but he was a good dad. Dads are more hands on these days, aren't they,' she pointed out, 'and I never felt I'd missed out.'

'Do you think that was because you were happier back then to take a secondary role as far as your work was concerned?'

'Oh yes,' Brenda said, 'you didn't expect to do as well as the men back then.'

'Was that a good thing?' I asked.

'I don't know, I've never really thought about it. But it's good for everyone to have choices.'

Brenda then went on to tell me about the couple next door to her where the woman earns more than her male partner. Brenda saw this as progress and her feminist side started to emerge. I asked her about seventies feminism. After all, Brenda was at her peak in 1971, being a comparatively young forty. It transpired that the seventies wave of feminism had not really touched her. She was aware of it but to her it was all about younger women who burnt their bras and had short hair. She really seemed to have just absorbed a caricature of seventies feminism and had not seen it as something for her. It has certainly been pointed out since, by some, that feminism back then tended to be for and about middle class, white, professionals. Brenda, who was older and came from a working class background, seemed to confirm this. I was pleased to be able to tell Brenda that the new wave of feminism today is keen to embrace all women and even has a word for it – intersectionality. There's no denying that an Asian girl concerned about FGM will have a different cause to fight than a forty year old woman trying to break the glass ceiling. But they both come under the same umbrella and there's a greater sense of everyone being in it together.

I asked Brenda whether she thought feminism could be important to her. And she told me IT WAS IMPORTANT TO ALL WOMEN. She said that she had felt her identity had been Geoff's wife and Robert and Wendy's mother. She felt sure that was changing and saw that as a good thing. 'Anything goes these days,' she said. 'I'd like to be young again.'

Wanting to be young again doesn't really fit in with one of the themes of this book so I tried to explain to her that she had a lot of experience to share with the world. She looked doubtful so I asked what was good about growing older.

'Nothing,' she said, 'I'm scared of being a burden to my children and I wonder what will happen if I lose my marbles.'

I felt rather despondent to hear about Brenda's fears. Brenda who had made the whole café laugh and who didn't seem to care what people thought of her as she banged her shopping bag into everything and wore whatever eccentric clothes she cared to. She proved it by ordering another cake, telling me it was too late to worry about her figure, eating half of it and then asking for a bag so she could take the other half home.

It seems to me that with feminism coming in waves, there are women where feminism has simply passed them by. I am pleased that new wave feminism is attempting to embrace all ages and sectors of society but we need to keep it going. We don't want a wave of feminism, we want a continuous waterfall which will leave a lasting effect. And as women live longer than men and our nursing homes are full of ageing women, then how we treat our old people is itself a feminist issue.

This chapter started by asking what we can learn from when our mothers were middle-aged. But we can also ask what we can learn from them now they are older. Of course, not all eighty year olds are like Brenda – feisty, determined, living life to the full. So perhaps my next list concerns what I have learnt from Brenda in particular.

1. Don't worry about what people think.
2. Look after your health. Being as mobile and healthy as you can will help you get the most out of life
3. Wear what the hell you like. (See point 1).
4. Mix with people of all ages. If you haven't got children or grandchildren, mix with someone else's.
5. Talk to people. Even to the staff in cafés.
6. Feminism concerns women of all ages.
7. Find out what you enjoy and do more of it.
8. Live each day as if it's your last. (Yes, that old mantra repeating itself). This gets steadily more important as you age.
9. Let the eccentric part of you emerge.
10. Smile. A smiling older person is as beautiful as a smiling baby.

Point ten has touched on an important issue for the middle-aged - beauty. Or what the older woman tends to see as fading beauty or lack of beauty. We have become a society increasingly concerned with what people look like. Part of me would like to dismiss this as trivial. I'd like to shout out at you all – IT DOESN'T MATTER WHAT YOU LOOK LIKE. But the problem is, it does to you. Because it really seems to matter to our society today. So much so it needs a whole chapter to itself.

THREE: THE WAY THINGS LOOK

There are three questions we need to ask about beauty. Firstly, why is beauty so important to women, secondly why do older women want to look younger and thirdly why has the focus for women become predominately about appearance so that women and girls feel constantly judged by what they look like? The balance is all wrong – in fact there really isn't any balance. Our greatest concern is for the younger generation because there is no doubt this is a rapidly growing problem and quite rightly this is being well documented and debated elsewhere. But to give one example, a report by the Girl Guides Association stated that a third of 11-14 year olds have stopped swimming or performing in school plays because they felt they were not attractive enough. What?! Seven out of ten of the girls surveyed felt they were judged more on looks than ability.

Sadly, body confidence is becoming an increasing problem in middle-aged women. A British Social Attitudes survey found that only 57% of women aged 35-49 are satisfied with their appearance. This seems to get slightly better as women get towards their older years but not much. In an interview with the Sunday Times in September 14, Jo Swinson, the equalities minister, blamed the growing number of older celebrities having plastic surgery and setting impossible standards. She also pointed out that the lack of older women in advertising and the media meant that women did not have normal examples of natural ageing reflected back to them. She criticised photo enhancing but praised some celebrities such as Emma Thomson who refuses to buy into the plastic surgery trend.

Women of all ages need to be concerned about the way things are going. Celebrities in their fifties are on the front of magazines air brushed out of all recognition. Sometimes the photo looks more like a small balloon with a few features painted on. What sort of message is this sending us? And if the young girls surveyed felt they were being judged on their looks, we now have to tell them that it doesn't get any better. UNLESS THINGS CHANGE.

Older women are revered for looking like younger women. It's as if their other achievements or their knowledge and wisdom are irrelevant details we needn't bother ourselves with. It's like saying - who cares if Rover can round up a flock of sheep, has saved his owner from drowning and been a life changing companion to an autistic boy, so long as his ears are in the right place.

Why is beauty so important to us and how has it become such a predominant need in our society that many would say has got out of hand? Here comes a touch of history, because the desire to look good has always been there. Stone Age people wore beads and painted their faces, much like a Neanderthal Adam Ant. Tribes, who have never had to endure advertisements where only beautiful people get the goods, still enhance themselves with jewellery and make up. Yes, even the tribal girl can't go out to the fireside till she's done her face. Interestingly when we look at the animal kingdom, it always seems to be the men going to the greatest lengths to lure in the opposite sex. The peahen looks like she hasn't made any effort while the peacock is giving it large with those feathers. (See also lions' manes, the antlers of a stag and the aptly named bird of paradise who has females swooning at him in a way even Justin Bieber would envy).

It's clearly all about sex. The animals make themselves look good and throw in a bit of a dance for good measure. A bit like us, I suppose. The purpose is to attract a member of the opposite sex to procreate. Though I don't advise giving that answer if you're in a night club and asked why you're wearing so much make up. But somehow it's all become a bit more than sex.

That being good looking is so important in life is sadly

undeniable. That it has an impact in everything we do, from what people think about us to the sort of job we are likely to get seems to be taking it too far. But research shows that your life is pretty well mapped out by how good looking you are. Studies have shown that neonatal nurses favour the better looking babies and teachers assume good looking children are also more intelligent and consequently give them more time than their uglier counterparts. It seems the beautiful have a head start in life.

For some reason, we accept this as chiselled in stone with no erase facility. We are told that good looking people have more opportunities so we think the best option is to make ourselves somehow become more good looking. Whatever that takes. And if that's not possible, then we think we must prepare ourselves for the worst job you can imagine. (Washing David Cameron's feet?). But it's like black women finding out they have a lower chance of getting a job somewhere so thinking the answer must be to make themselves whiter. No, no, no, no, no.

Instead of striving for perfect looks in our quest to 'achieve', WE NEED TO CHANGE ATTITUDES. Just as we have gone some way, at least, to changing attitudes about ethnic minorities, differing sexuality, and even women. With laws to help us. OK, there is still a way to go but progress has been made and no one has suggested that anyone should be less ethnic or less gay or not quite so disabled, for goodness sake. So we need to stop treating people differently according to their appearance. This is subtle so it's going to be harder, but it can be done. Teachers, for example, can be shown they have unconsciously ignored spotty Jenny with the wonky glasses in favour of a peach-skinned cute faced Samantha. And before all you teachers get defensive about this, as I said, it's unconscious. So let's make it conscious so that we can tackle our biases. So we start by drawing attention to the bias in favour of the beautiful so that IT CAN CHANGE.

Of course, we can't change nature – most women (though not all) will want to look good to attract a partner. Nothing wrong with that. Women also report that looking good boosts their confidence - they do it for themselves. This all sounds fine but EVERYTHING IN MODERATION. Looking as good as you can is not the same as chasing an impossible perfection we see flashed at us in the media. The middle path is the way in all things. So why not choose nice clothes that suit you and spend a little time doing your hair. But draw the line at a brand new face. Going out to a restaurant with mud all over your face and smelling of manure is not likely to either win you friends or help you feel good about yourself. But neither is staying in because a spot has appeared on your forehead you need a top of the range microscope to detect. Moderation. And doing what is both achievable and reasonable.

It could be argued that we associate beauty with youth and therefore older women want to be more beautiful as part of wanting to look and be younger. This all sounds like a sweeping generalisation, which it kind of is. Of course there are women who have no interest in looking younger and some who claim they have no interest in being good looking. And undoubtedly there is a certain freedom in that, provided it is not linked with an aspect of depression involving giving up on yourself. Many of us envy a clean, reasonably well groomed woman who has not placed her looks right at the top in her prioritisation. Who needs hang-ups about the minutiae of our appearance? But it's about finding what works for you. The truth is the vast majority of women want to be beautiful and the vast majority of older women say they would like to look younger. Is that quest for youth being dictated to us by the media, I wonder?

Women want to look good for very similar reasons, whatever their age. It may be to attract a partner, it will undoubtedly be to boost confidence and it may be to fit in with friends and society at large. Not many women would want to be the only person at a wedding in wellington boots, however damp the ground is outside the marquee. Many women enjoy dressing up and spending time on hair and makeup. Some may want to look a certain way at work to gain the confidence of their clients or customers. All well and good, but why do older women also want to look younger and is it the same thing?

We cannot deny that a part of the urge to look good might be to attract a mate. It's in nature. It's the way it is. And there has been a steady increase in the number of women in their fifties and sixties getting divorced and wanting to find love again. However, this still doesn't explain why these women want to look younger. The most likely reason is that in our society young is synonymous with attractive. And this assumption needs questioning. And changing. Beauty is surely ageless and timeless and so much more than counting wrinkles and grey hairs.

There are older role models available – women who have poise and charisma and are attractive WHILE LOOKING THEIR AGE. Judi Dench, Helen Mirren, Hilary Clinton, Meryl Streep. None of these, as far as I can tell, have had surgery. They simply MAKE THE MOST OF THEMSELVES. And that has to be a good thing. I personally find older women who have had a lot of surgical intervention very odd looking. As if they are constantly surprised to see you. Sorry, Anne Robinson, but I'm not the only one who finds it looks a bit, well, surgical. One problem is there are just not enough older women role models like the ones I've mentioned. Why? Because the majority of women on television are in their twenties and thirties. It's as if older women have been hidden away. Maybe there's a room somewhere in the vaults of the BBC or ITV where older presenters are waiting for a new TV which makes them look thirty years younger. OR A CHANGE IN ATTITUDE.

Of course the older women we do see are more often

than not victim to some cutting misogynous remarks. AA Gill who writes for the Sunday Times said he did not want to see historian Mary Beard on television seemingly because of her appearance. Never mind that she is an expert in her field and able to convey information in an accurate and interesting way. Female politicians are subject to criticisms of their appearance in a way their male counterparts are not. Older female presenters have been sidelined as they age, such as Miriam O'Reilly from Countryfile and Selena Scott. And television's loss of the wonderful Moira Stewart is Radio 2's gain. And yet we continue to adore the likes of David Attenborough, David Dimbleby and Tony Robinson giving no more than a passing thought to their age and appearance.

The message is clear. Women have a sell by date which men do not and to stay on television you have to be young or look young. I have some sympathy with Anne Robinson who felt she had to go the face lift route to remain on our screens, but really, does it make her any better at her job? Would we take less note of her reports on being swindled by the companies she features on Watchdog if she had a few more lines under her eyes? In the meantime, older women are getting the message loud and clear that to be anyone you need to look young or preferably be young. We need a much wider range of older role models from all spheres of life and where they are not subject to constant comments and criticism about their appearance. It's going to be a gradual change in attitude, but we can make a start.

I feel a to do list coming on:

1. If you particularly like an older female presenter then tell the BBC or whatever channel she appears on.
2. Campaign for having photo shopped photos of older women labelled as just that – altered.
3. Spread the word about achievements of older women and

campaign against newspaper columns entirely focused on their appearance.

4. Look at females (like the ones listed earlier) who make the most of themselves without going to ridiculous lengths to look younger. What do you want to look like – Helen Mirren or a Barbied fifty year old with boobs under her chin, a face that doesn't move and, most importantly, petrified in case a camera should catch her at a bad angle? There may be something in being allowed to dye and lift and tuck if that's what you want. But research has shown it rarely makes a woman happier. A woman who has not accepted her ageing and is paranoid about it, is nothing to aspire to.

5. If you are fifty five and look seventy, then yes, I can understand why you might want to look younger. But if you are fifty five and look fifty five, then hey, seems logical to me.

6. Think of all the things you have learnt to accept about yourself as you get older. I didn't like being one of the tallest in my class when I was thirteen. But I couldn't file my legs down so accepted it and now I love it. I accept that I am clumsy, that I can't sing, that I can't sew and so on. Just as I accept the things I can do. I am me. And you are you. I imagine if you've reached middle-age, you have also accepted your faults, strengths and weaknesses. So transfer that feeling to how you think about your looks.

7. Studies on happiness from all over the world have been collated by the World Happiness Database in Rotterdam. Sounds a wonderful place – I imagine Mary Poppins and the Cheshire Cat and The Laughing Policeman being in there somewhere. Anyway, research shows that you are happier if you THINK you are good looking rather than if you actually are. So, be confident about how you look by, well, building your confidence in general (more of this later, it's got a chapter of its own.)

8. Do not accept criticism for the way you look. As mentioned, AA Gill notoriously said historian, Mary Beard, should be kept away from the cameras all together, I surmise because of her appearance. Her responses were both clever and witty.

   She said Gill's paucity of learning may explain why he thinks he can pass off insult as wit. She joked that he should be made to watch all her programmes. And she said that even the greenest of her students would not present her with an essay as ill argued and off the point as Gill's critique. Job done. Beard clever and witty, Gill not.

9. Do not accept criticism like this directed at any older woman. Criticising or discriminating against anyone for being older, not traditionally attractive or just for being a woman is unacceptable. Don't accept it as normal, don't accept demeaning older women disguised as humour. If we are going to move towards respecting age and experience, then we should get rid of a culture where the opposite seems to be the case.

10. Find out what works for YOU. There is no such thing as a right or wrong way. Mary Beard is happy to let her grey hair be just that – grey hair. Nothing wrong with that. Helen Mirren has at the time of writing dyed her hair pink. Nothing wrong with that either. Appearance is primarily for confidence. As the research shows, it's about thinking you look good. Confidence is about being comfortable in your own skin. I don't feel comfortable in shorts or a mini skirt so I don't wear them. You might, so do. There are no rules about appearance here. Just check that you are dressing and altering your appearance for YOU and not for what you think is expected of you.

11. Lose the fear. Afraid of getting older? Then work on that fear. There is no cream that stops time passing. Having a face lift won't make you younger and so the fear will still be there.

12. Decide whose judgement you trust. If you trust your own judgement, then so much the better. But if you have a friend, partner, daughter or whoever to trust, get feedback from them. Someone honest to tell you if you look your best. We live in a judgemental society (see AA Gill) so gather people round you whose opinion you trust and then you can ignore anyone else.
13. Be selective about what magazines you buy and which journalistic columns you read.
14. If you don't give a flying fish what you look like, that's fine too.

Just a note on the last point. If you like to dress as a scarecrow, flaunt your hairy legs, grow a small beard and wear a plastic bag, then that's fine so long as you feel confident and empowered to do so. But ask yourself the following questions, just to check you are OK with your choice.

1. Do you want to fade into the background because you no longer feel you have anything to offer the world?
2. Do you think you are too old to bother about yourself? Maybe you think you've 'had your day.'
3. Do you want to make sure any sexuality you have (and we are sexual creatures well into our eighties and beyond) is hidden away?
4. Have you given up trying to look reasonable because you believe it's impossible at your age?
5. Do you feel down about life and yourself?

If you answered no to the above, then great – carry on being yourself. If you answered 'yes' to any of them, then you need to dig deep as you are making the scruffy choice for all the wrong reasons. You can be beautiful at any age and from any starting point.

OK, we really need to define beauty before we go any further. Let's start with what it isn't.

Beauty is NOT:-

Being under thirty.

Looking under thirty.

Being thin.

Being dressed in very expensive clothes.

Looking like the post op Anne Robinson.

Having good bone structure but looking miserable.

An exact science – there is no ideal height, weight, colouring.

Interesting without personality.

The same for everyone – there is considerable variation on who we find attractive.

Achievable through surgery.

Just about the physical.

ANYTHING AT ALL TO DO WITH AGE.

But beauty IS:

Found in confidence. (Research shows we rate confident people as more attractive).

Found in a smiling face.

Symmetry. (Research shows that all cultures favour a symmetrical face but hey, there are SO many exceptions).

In the eye of the beholder. (We fancy different people.)

Charisma.

Found in people of all ages.

Difficult to define.

As much about your soul as your body.

As much about your personality as your face.

Only one aspect of a human being.

Women and men who are more attractive earn more by between 10% and 20%. In Britain and the USA, we focus more on women's looks but in some cultures, such as Japan, China and Brazil, it is as much about men's looks as women's. And we most definitely associate good looks with youth in the Western world. Is this set in stone? Are we ever likely to revere those with larger than average noses or lust over ears that stick out? And is it ever possible to consider older people the most attractive? Maybe Prince Charles posters would then feature on all our bedroom walls for us to lust after.

Better than that would be to live in a world where looks are not as important as personality, contribution to society and, well, being a nice person. Age would therefore be unimportant when it came to judging looks, because we wouldn't be judging looks. But we know from the research that women are judged more on appearance than anything else and that older women are very likely to be passed over or ignored. Can that change? Well, one thing's certain, individual people can change their outlook. Take Dustin Hoffman.

At the time of writing, Hoffman's interview on being dressed as a woman for the film Tootsie is going viral. I remember reading soon after this film came out that a crew member had asked if he could introduce 'Dorothy' (the character Hoffman played) to a male friend to see if he noticed. The friend looked 'Dorothy' up and down and asked if he could see Jessica Lange. Hoffman began to realise that being a plain woman was hard going. Someone else he talked to while dressed as the character was clearly not listening to a word 'she' said because he was too busy looking around the room for someone more attractive.

In this more recent interview for AFI, Hoffman tells us more. He decided that he needed to look like a credible woman for the film to succeed. When he saw himself on film, he was disappointed he was not more attractive. He asked if he could be made more attractive but was told that it was as good as it gets. Maybe he instinctively knew that to be a woman, being attractive had become disproportionally important in society.

Then Hoffman had an epiphany. He went home to his wife and cried. This is what he said.

'I said to my wife, I have to make this picture and she said why and I said, because I think I'm an interesting woman when I look at myself on screen, and I know that if I met myself at a party, I would never talk to that character because she doesn't fulfil physically the demands that we're bought up to think that women have to have in order for us to ask them out. She said, what are you saying, and I said there are too many interesting women I have not had the experience to know in this life because I have been brain washed and....'

At this point, Hoffman pauses as he becomes emotional and adds, 'that was never a comedy for me.'

Hoffman's epiphany, when he realises that he MISSED OUT by focusing on women's looks is very moving. I imagine him now talking to women with equal interest whatever they look like and whatever their age. And if Hoffman, from the most looks orientated industry, can change so can others.

Interestingly Sir Tony Robinson, national treasure, has also come out and said that all men should dress in women's clothing for two years to show them a different way of thinking. This is all great stuff but a small part of me hopes that men are able to walk in our shoes more metaphorically. It might get very confusing out there if everyone looks like a woman. And they'd sell out of tights in M & S, most men being hopeless when it comes to wearing tights without laddering them. I happen to know that.

Research has shown that we have a fairly universal view of what physical beauty is – symmetrical face, symmetrical body and healthy appearance. Of course there are variations – the quirky looks where a bit of lopsidedness doesn't go amiss can be attractive to some. But let's go with the universal view of physical beauty for a moment. What happens to those women who fit this design when they get older? Surely, if you're born with symmetry, you keep it. Your nose doesn't suddenly twist to one side, or one ear shift up the side of your head a few inches. Do women actually lose their beauty? Well, no, they just lose their youth. And in this society, those who turned heads when they were younger seem to turn stomachs if they dare to age naturally. For some reason a few lines on your face, an inch or two around the stomach and fading hair colour renders you unattractive and unimportant. Time to change a few people's minds.

How do we get others to have a Dustin Hoffman style epiphany? We might not be able to change the world view of older women overnight, but we can start some ripples.

First, let's take a look at what we are up against.

1. Advertising campaigns that see youth as good, ageing as bad. Apparently we should all be buying anti ageing products because look, cream can actually stop you getting older. We are taken in by this false message even though NOTHING can stop us getting older (except death, which isn't really advertised at all, unless you count life insurance ads. Or that bingo ad which makes me want to end it all.) See also misleading slogans such as 'wrinkle repair' (really?), 'overnight repair' and my favourite – 'youth activating concentrate.' What increasingly annoys me are magazines which lure us in with feminist features which they print ALONGSIDE DEPICTING AN IDEALISED IMAGE OF AN OLDER WOMEN altered beyond realism.

2. There's been a recent spate of films featuring older people, looking about fifty but in old people's homes or with dementia or dying of cancer or generally having a miserable

time. Rare to see a sexually active, successful middle-aged person as a heroine we all aspire to be like. Middle-aged women are attractive. As middle-aged women. A recent survey by the UK film council found 60% of film goers questioned felt that older women were not portrayed as having any sexual desire. Yet we continuously see older male actors playing parts where they seduce women 20-30 years their junior. See also TV presenters where the current trend of older man and younger woman combination has almost become the norm. Let's reverse it. I'll happily volunteer to present alongside Harry Styles from One Direction.

3. Advertising campaigns which depict older women as stupid as well as unattractive. Take the German advert for Deutsche Bahn where an older woman hilariously knows how to book tickets on line to the surprise of everyone. Ha ha.

4. I have mentioned this before but cannot repeat it enough times, the double standard of middle-aged presenters on TV. Men can go on until they are carried away in a coffin, women are out at the first sign of a wrinkle.

5. Middle-aged men are admired for having a younger partner (as in shouting 'get in there!') Women are ridiculed for the same (as in desperate cougar). In fact the word cougar is problematic – firstly, there is no male equivalent suggesting it's only when the woman is older that it's worth labelling and commenting on. Secondly, it suggests predatory behaviour on the part of the woman.

6. There are far more older women on the radio suggesting it is their ageing looks that TV companies have trouble with. Miriam O'Reilly, the 53 year old Countryfile presenter who successfully sued the BBC for age discrimination was told nine months before she was sacked to be 'careful with those wrinkles when high definition comes in.' Some women have become successful on the radio having been mostly dropped

on TV, such as Vanessa Feltz and Moira Stewart.

7.   We are also up against Gillitian views.

We can summarise quite simply by stating the bleeding obvious – women are more judged on their looks than men. And middle-aged women are often considered past their sell by date purely based on their so-called fading looks. Our society fails to see that women can be attractive at any age and that attraction is far more than just waist size x smooth skin x youthful hair colour. To a great extent, middle-aged women have become invisible – on our screens, on the stage, in advertising.

There are signs of a slight shift. Since Miriam O'Reilly-gate, the BBC has acknowledged the need for older presenters. Films portraying older women got off to a bad start using death as the main theme but It's Complicated starring Meryl Streep and Cedar Rapids with Sigourney Weaver are exceptions which may set a new trend. Adverts for anti ageing products are getting the ridicule they deserve, as are men like Godfrey Bloom (more about this ridiculous man and others like him later).

Best of all is Dustin Hoffman's epiphany. It can't just be Hoffman who's re-thought the less traditionally attractive woman. It can't just be David Dimbleby and John Humphries who have recognised the need for older women in the media (yes, they've said it). It can't just be me who is horrified at the combination of ageism and sexism that seems acceptable. Although to be fair, I know nobody who agrees with AA Gill about Mary Beard. Or about anything, for that matter. Though let's give him some credit – he can write well.

FOUR: WRITTEN AND UNWRITTEN LAWS

There are laws against discrimination concerning age. There are also sexual discrimination laws. So older women must be treated equally. So there. But are the laws working? Let's look at what they are first. In 2010 the spanking new, all singing, all dancing equality act bought together all the existing regulations into one big one. A bit like The Spice Girls, The Supremes, Girls Aloud, Bananarama and The Bangles joining forces into one all encompassing girl band. On paper, it should work but what about the reality?

The law protects against ageism in employment, education and training. This includes universities, clubs, associations and trade bodies. Added to that, since 2012, people can expect equal and fair treatment when receiving goods and services, whatever their age. Discrimination falls into four categories – direct, indirect, harassment and victimisation. Bear with me - this really is worth getting your head round.

Direct discrimination is where you are discriminated against directly. Obviously. Such as not being promoted simply because your employer thinks you're past it. You know the sort – arranges the works outing in a night club and just assumes any staff over forty-five will prefer to stay at home with an Ovaltine and a box of chocs. So when it comes to promotion, you've got as much chance as the Queen being break dance champion of the world.

Indirect discrimination is where it is implied older people are not welcome. Job adverts which ask for recent graduates. Or states that people who remember the Beatles need not apply.

Harassment is behaviour which makes you feel intimidated or degraded or that creates a hostile environment because of your age. Or indeed someone associated with you – so constant jokes about your age or your partner's age. Now, there are grey areas here (unintentional pun). I sometimes make jokes about my age. But a boss who constantly undermines you with annoying jokes meant to belittle you is another thing altogether. I doubt, as well, that it would be worth suing the young sales assistants who raise their eyebrows when you dare to venture into Topshop. (Although that's a pity).Of course I don't think we want to ban all funny comments about age but the purpose of them, their intention, needs looking into. And I personally believe that you should be able to sue anyone who thinks they are funny but are not.

Victimisation is where you are treated unfairly as a result of making a complaint about ageism. Yours or someone else's. So if you back Sandra from the office when she complains about being called an old bag in meetings by Nigel, Nigel can't then get his own back by demoting you to a position where you have to clean his shoes.

Of course ageism applies to the young as well. It is illegal to discriminate against anyone because of their age and that applies to all generations. This is rarer but certainly there have been cases where a woman has been told she was too young for the job, assuming she was less capable than an older woman. Of course, where there is an objective justification for employing a person of a certain age, then that's fine. So I won't be auditioning for the part of teenage girl in Hollyoaks then.

When you read the details of the law, many of you will be thinking about your particular Nigel in the office who enjoys those ridiculous ageist comments. He'll be the same Nigel who likes to make sexist comments too. The Nigel who is probably secretly hung up about his lack of success with women. By the way, all Nigels out there, I only picked the name Nigel at random. He could just as easily be called Adrian Anthony (or AA, for short). So what to do about it?

1. Some (only a few) men are so stupid, they genuinely think they are funny. Or they really don't know they are being sexist and/or ageist. So start by just explaining to them why you feel offended or discriminated against. Calmly. Avoid shouting it out at the water dispenser in front of everyone, thus humiliating him back again. HOWEVER BAD HIS COMMENTS. He may genuinely not realise how annoying he is being. He probably thinks he's hilarious. So to start with at least give him a chance to put it all right himself. Ask him to join you for coffee or make an appointment to see him privately. Whatever's appropriate to the situation. Explain that he has made you feel annoyed/belittled/discriminated against and ask him to cease his jokes, comments or actions.

2. If this doesn't work, present him with the legalities. Say that on behalf of all older women, you would be prepared to take it further but that you don't really want to (although maybe you do.)

3. If it doesn't stop, contact HR. This is on behalf of all older women, so do it. No point whinging to your mates, TAKE ACTION.

4. At each stage, keep calm. Nothing worse than the usual sexist male retort of 'Don't get hysterical.'

5. If he does say that, then you might as well get hysterical so consider either kicking him in the testicles or spreading rumours about his small penis.

6. Actually, I don't advocate the above. No point fighting against inappropriate remarks with inappropriate remarks of your own. (So don't worry AA Gill, I'm not going to mention you again. Probably.)

7. If you have a successful case of age discrimination, share it with the world. This will alert everyone to this law and how it can be applied. You may prevent someone else from experiencing this sort of behaviour.

The most important point here is not to accept discrimination against yourself either as an older person or as a woman or both. The other important point to make is DON'T DISCRIMINATE AGAINST YOURSELF either. This needs some explanation.

1. Ever catch yourself thinking or saying – 'I'm too old to...' Well take a step back and say 'Who says so?' You are not too old to go for that promotion – even the law agrees with you. And you are not too old to bungee jump/wear a bikini/sleep in a tent at Glastonbury/change careers/build sandcastles. Maybe, like me, you don't want to bungee jump. That's fine. Just check it's not because someone has told you you're too old or that society has set a culture where we think we're too old to do things.

2. Don't hold back. Go for a promotion if you want to. Good clichés to use are 'never too late' and 'a change is as good as a rest' and 'life begins now.' Clichés are overused because there's some truth to them.

3. Don't get any set notions about age and health. You can be twenty seven and fall ill. Just because you're heading towards sixty doesn't mean you are counting the years towards ill health. There is a law now against being forced to retire. Keep going as long as you want to.

4. There are no laws dictating how you have to behave at any age (except those under eighteen things, but we needn't bother about that now.)

5. One more cliché – age is just a number. Actually that's not completely true. Age is just the number of years' useful experience you've had.

I don't want to put a dampener on things, but the number of sex discrimination laws brought about by employees has fallen by 80% since the law changed in 2013. This may be because employees are expected to fork out up to £1,200 to take their employer to tribunal. The TUC are not impressed and would like this to change. There is financial help for those that need it but my understanding is that when this is calculated, the woman's (or man's) partner's income is taken into account and only a very few qualify. Sometimes the union will put up the money and I know unions are trying to change things as I write. The other dampener I am going to throw at you is that only a small percentage of discrimination cases (and that is all discrimination) succeed. Usually because of lack of evidence so make sure you document everything if you think you are heading this way. End of dampeners, pour yourself a large glass of wine and continue. It will get more positive again. Eventually.

Retirement Law

Just a quick note about the current laws on retirement. Generally, you have the right to retire any time so long as you are able to do the job. There are some exceptions such as if you are in the police or fire brigade but mostly, you decide. However, there are all sorts of grey areas and exceptions. For example in 2012, a lawyer was forced to retire at 65 as it was reasonable for younger employees to become a partner after a certain amount of time.

You can go on the GOV.UK website to work out the age you can take your state pension which for most women will be 66. And you can now take a quarter of your private or company pension out at 55. I am not going to dish out any financial advice on this but would recommend you take some from an expert.

If laws are there, we need to make sure everyone is aware of them and that they are used and enforced when necessary. One example of a law which is not being used fully at the time of writing is the law against FGM (female genital mutilation). This has been banned since 2003 but with a conservative 66,000 women in the UK living with it and 20,000 girls under fifteen at risk of FGM, where are the arrests? It is also illegal to arrange for a girl to travel abroad to have this barbaric act carried out. This is clearly child abuse and CONCERNS US ALL so I wanted to give it a quick mention as one of the most urgent of all feminist issues. The law is there and yet it is not enough without some action. The same goes for all laws. USE THEM.

We've touched on the law and we've begun to touch on those unwritten laws – telling us we have to behave in a certain way in keeping with our age. We're even expected to look a certain way – younger than our years (see previous chapter). If you've ever felt awkward in some settings or situations simply because of your age, then you may have inadvertently come across one of these unwritten laws. The best way to tackle these is to stick together. Safety in numbers. Grey (or chestnut brown tinged/ natural blonde enhanced) power. Middle-aged masses.

You are not alone and neither am I. In the UK, over twenty million people are aged fifty and over – a third of the total population. And more than half of them are women. Back in 2008, people aged 60 and over outnumbered children (the under sixteens) for the first time. In the United States, by 2050 forty percent of the population will be over fifty. We are getting older so statistically, the youth should not be dictating anything. Yet they do.

Not that I am suggesting the older generation take over in some sort of coup. I'm not looking to lock up Little Mix and One Direction and not let them out until they hit forty or Cilla Black/Cliff Richard has passed away (whichever happens first). I'm not looking to kick our young politicians out of parliament and encourage Prince William to retire before he's even started the job. I'm not planning on campaigning that the age of consent needs pushing up to forty-one. It's not about older women being more important than anyone else (although, I'd be tempted by that particular campaign) it's about getting rid of discriminatory views. It's about EQUALITY. It's about a society that does not make negative judgements about someone just because she's a woman and she's middle-aged.

Middle-aged women are not some sort of minority group, even if we are made to feel like it. We have our age range and our gender in common but that's about all. We all come from different backgrounds, some of us are disabled, we may have differing sexuality, we may have different views on any manner of things. BUT WE NEED TO JOIN TOGETHER TO MAKE SURE WE HAVE A VOICE. Just because there are lots of us doesn't mean there's no discrimination. Look at women in general and read the postings on the everyday sexism project. You'd think there were way more men in the world. Now add age into the equation and we have a problem. We are feeling sidelined and unimportant. And if you don't feel represented, listened to and respected you can quickly lost your confidence.

Let's sweat the small stuff first. There are places where we are certainly not banned like some sort of grey apartheid, but where we feel, well, awkward. Equally, there are places where middle-aged or older people dominate and this feels slightly wrong too. I wonder whether it all goes back to our schooldays where we are all put in classes with others of exactly the same age. Years ago when women tended to do things at similar times, we still seemed a bit stuck in age groups. So undergraduates, newly weds, new mums, grandmothers were all reaching milestones at roughly the same age. But times have changed. Universities and colleges are full of people of all ages, new mothers cover a much wider age spectrum, and we retire at any time from fifty five to ninety five. Gone are the nineteen forties and fifties where you could find offices full of young typists who immediately left when they got married to be replaced by more young typists.

Now we are more likely to work in mixed age groups

61

and have friends of different ages. Studies have shown that we tend to have friends at the same STAGE of life as us but this could be ten or fifteen years apart. Or more. And then there are the later dating groups. With more divorce, more people putting off a long term relationship until later in life and more middle-aged people looking for a new love, we suddenly have a much more diverse group of people at the 'looking for love' stage. This is all great, as far as I'm concerned. Suddenly, we are more mixed up socially – bars and clubs are more likely to have mixed aged groups, younger girls are now getting into craft circles and the women's institute, student unions are full of all ages, and rock concerts have very diverse audiences – an audience watching the Rolling Stones will be a mix of new young fans and those who remember them when they started. Similarly, I have not felt out of place watching new music acts.

Personally, I don't like going to activities aimed at a particular age group – I like the mix, but I can see there are some occasions where a narrower age range might be popular. Over forties nights at night clubs, for example, where the music is likely to be chosen to include some memory joggers and where the environment is right for women who are choosing to try and meet a partner of a similar age. I can see that there may be self help groups attracting a very defined age range (menopausal support groups are unlikely to be full of teenagers). However, there are still some places and situations where a middle-aged or older person might feel unnecessarily awkward or unwanted. This to me is a shame. And it's probably got far more to do with lack of confidence than not being welcomed. For example, if you go into a shop which sells fashions aimed at the young, I doubt very much that you will be unwelcome, especially if you have a credit card about your person, but we can feel, well, awkward. With a society that tends to favour the young and ignore women past a certain age, it is all too easy to feel you have no worth, no right to be here, no voice to be heard. We will allocate a whole chapter to confidence, but in the mean time, get support from your same age friends and colleagues and do the following, if you want. You can do them on your own of course, but being in a group might be better for anyone lacking confidence and will certainly be better if you're wanting to make a stand.

1. Go to any high street store that seems to cater for younger shoppers. A pair of jeans doesn't change just because you've hit forty or fifty. And don't pretend you're shopping for your daughter.
2. Visit any bar or club that takes your fancy. And don't pretend you're in there looking for your daughter.
3. Dress young, dress old, dress like a banana. Ignore fashion advice that says older people should wear certain styles. IT'S UP TO YOU.
4. Ignore any advice to older women which contains the words 'should' or 'ought to.'
5. Talk to people of all ages. There's no law which says you have to seek out people of your age. Or even your stage. Take an interest in issues which affect other age groups – uni fees, care homes, child care costs etc. Then get talking.
6. Take up whatever sport or activity you want to take up. No rule that says you can't. Do it.
7. Take a gap year. This doesn't just apply to the late teens who have just left school. It applies to anyone – particularly popular for parents who have just emptied their nest.
8. I once attended a writing forum for under thirties. They couldn't stop me and I made a point. Do something similar if you feel like it.
9. If you feel judged or awkward, say so. It may just be in your head or someone might need to change their mind about you.

10. Dance as if nobody's watching. Sing as if no one can hear. Express yourself in whichever way you want – whether it's through what you wear, what you say, what you write, how you move. Be the person you want to be in the place you want to be in, with the people you want to be with.

I would like to add another rule – use humour. Learn how to make a witty retort, learn how to laugh at yourself and don't take life in your middle-age too seriously. This is more important than you think and deserves a chapter all of its own.

FIVE: YOU'RE HAVING A LAUGH

Sexism, ageism and particularly both together is serious stuff. It affects us all and creates the sort of society no one really wants. Even those who think they want it. But recently, feminism has used humour to good effect to make some valid points. Seventies feminism made some fantastic strides in the right direction, women's roles were questioned and widened, laws were changed, and feminism did its job in bringing attitudes into the twentieth century. There are some criticisms being bandied about now suggesting it had all been too earnest and angry. I think it was probably what was right for the time. And what seems to be working now, in the twenty first century, is a more witty and inclusive feminism.

I warmed to the women in moustaches breaking into boardrooms to draw attention to the lack of females getting through that glass ceiling. And take a look at the humorous feminist photographs by Sarah Marple. Enjoy the wit of the writing from new feminist icons such as Caitlin Moran. Feminist groups, writing and campaigns are now all laced with a healthy dose of satire, irony and sarcasm. And I love it. It just feels right for today. It's a new wave and it's important that we don't just recreate what's gone before even if some of the messages are the same. So I won't be throwing myself under a horse at the Derby then. Unless I can think of a witty retort to shout out as I go under. Something about burgers, maybe.

Of course, twinning wit and feminism is nothing new. You only have to read Dorothy Parker or Jane Austen. And even 1970s feminists had a few laughs along the way. With angry and radical undertones naturally. But what about femi-ageism? (Ooh, I may have invented a new word!) Can we laugh as we are attacked for daring to be a middle-aged woman? Yes, I think we can. Of course, this is not to be confused with jokes told by the likes of Les Dawson, jokes which simply reinforce stereotypes of older females. This is about lightening up to make a serious point.

The serious point is that older women are often sidelined in society, made to feel invisible, being written off too soon, discriminated against for being older AND for being a woman. But if I wrote all that on a placard or in a pamphlet, I'm not sure I'd exactly be changing the world. We need humour for a number of reasons.

1. We need humour in life anyway. Laughter got me through cancer – that's how vital it is.
2. We need it to make people listen and take notice. That means being creative with how we get the message across. Anyone trying to influence others will contemplate using humour – just look at any advertising campaign. Or political satire – some claim good satire can bring governments down.
3. The best way to show how out of date some attitudes are is to poke fun at them. I can see it now – a sketch with men patronising an I.T. consultant, assuming she can't understand technology. Another sketch with people looking around a room full of middle-aged women, pretending they can't see anyone. No? I'll stick to writing books then. There are others far more experienced at satire than I am to challenge those stereotypes in a humorous way. I could poke fun at Godfrey Bloom, I suppose. But then he makes his attitudes look ridiculous all on his own.
4. Getting angry with the frustration of it all invites comments to make us even angrier (Calm down, dear. Why do women get so hysterical? Are you on your period? Menopausal?) These comments are designed to wind us up, so don't let them.
5. So have some retorts ready for those irritating comments.

Meet inappropriate unfunny jokes about your age with inappropriate unfunny jokes about the size of his penis. Or preferably something wittier.

6. Unfortunately, many older women have reported that other women are sometimes the ones making ageist comments, about appearance in particular. Mutton dressed as lamb, what does she think she looks like etc. This seems particularly unnecessary but, when you think about it, not that important. Laugh off the small stuff and concentrate on what really matters.

7. The menopause is a natural stage of life and yet no one likes to talk about it. It's become something ever so slightly embarrassing, like noticing your skirt tucked into your knickers or farting in a meditation class. Laugh about it. Tell everyone you're just taking a personal journey to the tropics. Announce that you've never known a February as hot as this one. By laughing at it, you give everyone permission to talk about it. You've bought it out into the open and that's good.

8. Laughing at sexist and ageist comments ridicules them. You might even persuade the person who uttered them to laugh too. Saying – do you realise what you've just said – and then laughing at it, might open up a light hearted discussion about how you feel.

9. Laughing is SO much better than crying when it comes to sexist ageism. Crying only provokes those period/menopause comments anyway.

10. It's all about balance. Yes, we should get angry if we are passed over for promotion because of our age. But using humour alongside anger and, more importantly, action, can only strengthen your argument.

So when is something funny, or more often something meant to be funny, just downright misogynous? If we don't laugh at a joke about middle-aged/menopausal women are we displaying a sense of humour bypass? I think we usually just KNOW when something is humorous and when something is an insult disguised as humour. Women have a real intuition for these things. Firstly, we can tell what the intention of the 'joker' is and secondly if it's not insulting and we laugh at it easily and without feeling uncomfortable, then it tends to be all right.

There are occasional events or jokes which divide us, however. Take Halloween 2013 when Heidi Klum dressed as an elderly woman with varicose veins, liver spots, grey hair and a walking stick. There then followed a column in the Guardian suggesting this was depicting ageing women in a negative and stereotypical way. Was it meant to be ironic, funny, making a point about society or, as the Guardian columnist suggested, in rather bad taste and doing nothing for older women? That's why I wrote we USUALLY know. You decide on this one. It didn't make me laugh, it didn't make me uncomfortable, it just made me think there are better Halloween costumes. There are other examples of course such as Jeremy Paxman joking that there are too many old people and so there should be a Dignitas on every corner disguised as a tea shop. Vaguely amusing I suppose but be careful what you wish for, Jeremy (64 when he said this, maybe in a 'tea shop' by the time you read this).

I sometimes joke about certain aspects of getting older to cope with them so might, for example, find myself laughing to friends about how I had a senior moment and put my car keys in the fridge. The only problem with this is it can turn into some sort of competition as to who has the funniest memory loss story. 'You put your car keys in the fridge - that was nothing, I lost my car in a car park' followed by 'car lost - trivial, I forgot who I was for a good hour.' I feel a Monty Python sketch is waiting to be written. I even found myself talking to an old friend recently who claimed to be hotter than me (as in hot flush, not ability to pull).

We ended up laughing hysterically at this competitive menopause syndrome. And that made us even hotter.

As attitudes change, so humour changes. This doesn't mean we have LESS humour in our society. I remember a time when you could switch on your television and see the likes of Jim Davidson and Bernard Manning telling racist, homophobic and sexist jokes which people seemed to laugh at. When you hear them now, they quite rightly make you cringe. This doesn't mean you can't have jokes which feature black or gay people – they just have to be FUNNY. And being funny means NOT buying into stereotypes or ridiculing people just because of their race, religion, sexuality or gender. Or age. People get very confused about this but it's really quite simple – if a joke or funny remark makes you feel uncomfortable, then there's something not quite right. If a joke's only funny if that woman/Irishman/Muslim is not in the room then beware. You CAN tell jokes about black people – listen to Lenny Henry, you CAN tell jokes based on being gay – see Julian Clary. But they all have something important in common – they are quite often POKING FUN at stereotypes and outdated attitudes. Or they are simply rejoicing in their colour or sexuality in a way which brings a smile to all our faces.

What about female comics? I have one thing to say – YAY JO BRAND. Oh and Victoria Wood, French and Saunders, Jenny Eclair and so many more. As I discovered when writing the above paragraph, you can't easily analyse humour. I tried dissecting some jokes but this has one result – it immediately prevents the joke from being funny. And as I said, you just know when a joke about an older woman is funny and when it's insulting - it will either make you laugh or make you want to punch the comic in the face.

The funny women I've mentioned are all getting a little older now. So they are also great role models of women we DO sit up and take notice of. YAY Jo Brand for making us laugh at periods when some people still think they can't be mentioned. And Victoria Wood for the funny stuff about your hysterectomy. And all women who make us see that getting older is funny in the most joyful way. Periods, menopause, hysterectomies, vaginal problems and, heaven's above, women masturbating – women's issues which have become taboo. Why? Because men, in particular, don't want to have to think about any of it. Probably because they were spoken about in hushed tones by their mothers. And some of those topics (menopause, hysterectomies) specifically concern older women. So please, you great female (and indeed male) comedians - none of these subjects should be taboo. When they are tackled in a sexist or ageist way, maybe that's taboo. But not the topics themselves.

There is also the matter of laughing at yourself. Comedy comes from experience. Which is why Lenny Henry can be funny talking about the experience of being a black man in Cornwall. And Alan Carr can talk about being a gay son of a football manager with great mirth. (Whereas Jim Davidson was simply racist and homophobic in my opinion) And so if Jenny Eclair laughs about getting older, then the comedy has some truth to it. Which makes it all the funnier. We identify with her. We laugh with her. And we can do it too. Laugh at ourselves but without stereotyping all older women.

Enough about humour. We're British. We're funny. We do satire and irony better than anyone. Use it. Enjoy it. Whatever your age and gender. But in my experience, middle-aged women who have managed to retain their confidence and self-esteem, are the wittiest of all. Celebrate it.

SIX: THE VOICE IN YOUR HEAD

If the voice in your head is saying 'I am completely happy with who I am, I embrace getting older, I have the confidence not to let my age or sex get in the way of anything, I live life to the full and I'm an all round good egg,' then skip this chapter. But if you're a woman over forty, then this is unlikely. In fact, research shows that if you're a woman of any age this is unlikely.

Summarising all the research in my own way, it seems a man is more likely to think 'I can go for any job I want,' while a woman is more likely to say 'Not sure I'm good enough for that promotion.' A man is likely to see a good looking man in the mirror (even when his stomach hangs over like he's got a walrus stuffed up his jumper) whereas a woman is likely to see a woman with a hideous deformity by way of a nose the size of Concorde or a bottom the size of Devon (even if she's a well paid model).

Of course I am falling into the trap of making sweeping generalisations about the sexes – there are obviously confident women and there are men who lack confidence but the trend has been proved. It seems it is lack of confidence which is a huge factor in holding women back. Girls are doing way better than boys at all levels of education, getting better exam results at school and making up more than 60% of graduates. And yet, it's the men who are nabbing all the top jobs. But more telling, IT'S THE MEN WHO BELIEVE THEY CAN GET THE TOP JOBS and so it's the men who apply, with all the self belief of Simon Cowell in a Simon Cowell look alike competition.

Women have a tendency to underestimate their abilities. Researchers from UCL analysed thirty studies into gender issues in 2008 and found that men are not cleverer than women (you don't say) but that they think they are. For example, women underestimate their IQs by an average of 5 points. Men don't. They are more likely to overestimate. Another study asked men and women in a workforce to apply for a fictitious manager's post. Even women with the right qualifications and experience to apply doubted their ability, whereas men were generally more likely to think they could do the job, including a male office junior with no relevant qualifications. No wonder men earn, on average, 10% more than women.

The Dove campaign of 2013 asked women to describe themselves for an artist to draw and then asked other women to describe her. The pictures drawn where the woman had described herself were sadder and less attractive than when someone else had described her. It's not looking good for women's self-confidence, is it?

Lack of confidence in all women is not just about appearance and work promotions. It can and will affect all aspects of life. I recently took part as an audience member on Question Time. A member of the production team phoned me and asked me if my husband and I had questions we wanted to ask. I explained that we both had different questions to put forward. She seemed relieved and during the course of the conversation, told me that there were many women, particularly older women, who would say that they were just coming with their partner and didn't want to say anything. WHY GO ON QUESTION TIME IF YOU DON'T HAVE A BURNING QUESTION? You might as well go for a swim at the pool with no intention of getting wet. It seems that there are still a large number of women who just sit back on programmes such as this, hoping someone else (a man, presumably) will ask the question they want answered. It's back to the school room where boys are more likely to put up their hands than girls. I am told it's the same on quiz programmes such as Who Want To Be A Millionaire, where there are many more male applicants. Women, it seems, are more likely to have a fear of failure or a fear of making a fool of themselves. Men seem happy to take the risk.

And it's by taking risks and sometimes failing that we eventually succeed.

Although women are more likely to lack the confidence to push themselves forward in the workplace and elsewhere, the good news is SELF CONFIDENCE AND SELF ESTEEM CAN CHANGE. And at any age. It's never too late to boost your confidence and change your outlook.

Older women seem to be even more susceptible to low self esteem and lack of self-belief perhaps because they grew up in a time when men were even more dominant in the workplace, in sport, well everywhere. And if older women are not given a strong voice in society, then this isn't going to do anything to help. Let's have a list of why women's self esteem is at risk and why older women have it bad. For all women:

1. They are very likely to have been ridiculed by men at some point in their life. There are misogynist comments in the air. Just go to a football match and listen to some of the chants (you play like a girl etc).

2. Recent twitter and internet trolling has been focused on women and tends to criticise them or their appearance rather than their point of view. Yes, when it comes to twitter abuse on women, it gets personal.

3. Research shows that girls at school are more likely to be praised for being good and writing neatly. A certain amount of 'pushiness' and questioning authority is expected from boys. So they just get more practice at acting confidently.

4. There are many aspects of life where men have succeeded ahead of women. Sportsmen get more TV coverage and pay than women, for example, and the same goes for stand up comedy. We seem to expect men to be better at some things just because of past traditions.

5. Women are different neurologically, with stronger language

centres, for example. It's likely then that women do more self evaluation and therefore more self criticism. While men just get on with it.

6. An old boys' network still exists out there. When women are excluded from this, it doesn't do much to help their confidence.

7. Women are judged for the wrong things. A female politician who makes a good speech must wonder if she has, in fact, made a good speech when the only comments made are to do with her hair, weight, or colour of her handbag.

8. A survey by Peugeot in 2012 found 57% of men lack confidence so maybe we just show it more. (Though to be fair, the same survey showed many more women than that lacked confidence – about 2 out of 3.)

9. A Yougov survey commissioned by the Sunday Times found that 82% of women, against 73% of men had never asked their employer for a promotion. And nearly twice as many men as women had asked their employer for a pay rise. And yet 34% of women surveyed thought they were MORE capable of doing the job than those senior to them. One in five of the women blamed a lack of self confidence. Sylvia Ann Hewlett, a British economist, suggested women chose the wrong sort of mentor – one who could be a friend rather than someone in a position of power who might help them up through the hierarchy.

So we all lack confidence some of the time, young or old, male or female. (Though older women seem to be more at risk than most.) Where it becomes a problem is when it prevents us from reaching our potential or from simply being happy. But there's some good news. Hooray. It concerns the younger generation. Oh. A study from the University of Basel based on surveys of 7,100 young people found that young women had just as much confidence as men. Hooray. But that seems to contradict the Peugeot survey. Oh. Maybe it depends which car you drive.

Head teachers of all girls schools certainly seem to think younger women lack more confidence than their male counterparts (stay with me, this is going to be relevant to older women. Eventually.) In 2012, girls from Wimbledon High School were taught boasting, self promotion and celebrating success as part of a 'Blow your own trumpet' week. And Putney High school are proposing to teach sixth formers improvised comedy and stand up in order to teach risk taking and thinking on your feet, all part of self-confidence. We will think on these activities when we discuss how older women can boost their self confidence. The interesting point is that all these things from self-promotion to stand up comedy are all things men tend to be good at. OK, not all men can do stand up and be funny. Not all stand up comics can do stand up and be funny, come to think of it. But you get my drift. WE CAN LEARN ABOUT SELF CONFIDENCE FROM MEN AS WELL AS CONFIDENT WOMEN. More of that later.

Let's get back to older women and why they, more than other women, are likely to lack self-confidence.

1. In a society that still seems to judge a woman on her looks and places a great emphasis on youth, it's hard to maintain confidence in your appearance as you age.
2. Older women often feel apologetic for being older. Like it's their fault. Many of us suffer from 'failed-to-be-young syndrome.'
3. An older woman may have gained self-confidence from her role in bringing up the children. After all, it's no easy task and many are proud to have carried it out successfully without the aid of a vat of gin and small warehouse of fags. When the children fly the nest, some of a woman's self worth

can disappear.

4. They may feel threatened at work by a new generation of high flyers biting at their ankles.
5. They will probably have been bought up in a time when men were expected to be more successful than women.
6. Older women are simply less revered by most of our society.

OK, I seem to be painting a picture of a nation of quivering older women hiding behind their mother's gravestone and not wanting to come out and face the world. Some older women are more confident than others but the point is OLDER WOMEN ARE AT RISK OF LOSING THEIR CONFIDENCE. And we need to do something about it.

Interestingly, studies have found that where women are self confident, they have a slightly different self-confidence than men. Men tend to have a self-confidence based on how they perform tasks which will include doing well at work and winning at sport. Women, on the other hand, tend to have a self-confidence based on more personal traits such as integrity and compassion. We feel more confident if we believe we are perceived as better people.

But the outcome to being confident, in whatever form, is being comfortable in our own skin.

Being confident is NOT:
1. Telling the funniest joke in the loudest voice.
2. Always being the one to start the Conga going (whether at the office party or just on a Saturday morning in Tesco's.)
3. Being absolutely certain that everything you say is right.
4. Being absolutely certain that everything anyone else says is wrong.
5. Knowing that Simon Cowell is completely misguided when he says your rendition of 'I will survive' was out of tune,

because you know you have the X factor in shovel loads.

Being confident IS:
1. Being happy and confident with who you are, right now.
2. Having a realistic self belief which enables you to have a go at whatever you want to.
3. Not imagining everyone is looking at you, but not minding if they are.
4. Knowing your viewpoint is valid.
5. Never being afraid to say 'I don't know' and to ask questions.

Is there such thing as over confidence? It could be argued that the banking and financial crises in recent years were all caused by over confidence. In fact, there is more danger to the world from over confidence than under confidence. Over confidence can mean putting all caution aside and behaving recklessly. And over confidence can mean arrogance. Now, we have to be a bit careful about arrogance. Of course we've all met a truly arrogant person (look how I've carefully avoided saying man). The sort whose self belief has tipped over into thinking their view and their view alone is all that counts, the sort that thinks they are literally God's gift to woman/man and that anyone who disagrees is gay/blind/stupid/in denial. We've all seen the out of tune wimp on programmes such as X factor who looks aghast and in complete disbelief when told they haven't got any sort of factor at all, not even a personality, nothing. Their conclusion? Simon Cowell doesn't know what he's talking about. Presumably the millions he's made has just been a bit of luck then. But sometimes we come across the sort of arrogance which is just a defence mechanism. A very unconfident person over compensating for their lack of confidence by putting on a bad act. And if you are one of those people, you need to be brave enough to show your vulnerability. Admit to a lack of confidence and people will warm to you. And that's a start.

Which brings me to outer confidence and inner confidence. It's inner confidence we need but we might need to start with outer confidence to get us going. Let me explain. Confidence is not really how you behave on the outside. We can envy the woman who walks into a party, goes up to a stranger, looks him in the eye and introduces herself with a witty one liner. I've done that. I've also been shaking inside when I've done it. I've also had a couple of glasses of wine before doing it. I've also gone on to the next person and said something stupid, shattering the confidence I had just about mustered. Sometimes it's the quieter person listening to someone, asking questions, putting her opinion in careful succinct sentences who is the most confident. She's confident on the inside and doesn't need to prove it with jokes and presenting a big personality to the waiting world. Of course it varies from person to person and it's hard to judge who has that inner confidence. We're all different.

However, outer confidence can turn into inner confidence. On those occasions, when you do that walking into the room, witty introduction thing, any good response you receive inevitably boosts your inner confidence. In fact, just doing it boosts your inner confidence. And that in turn means you get better at the outer confidence. Staying away from the party or turning up and hiding in the kitchen with the gin will simply reinforce your lack of confidence. You don't need to be the life and soul of the party – that might just be outer confidence anyway. But if you turn up, enjoy it and interact as much or as little as feels good to you, then you've been one confident woman.

It's also not as simple as being either confident or unconfident. Many women are confident in familiar situations but not so confident in unfamiliar surroundings or situations. This is perfectly understandable. It's no bad thing to be cautious, to feel your way with people and places. However, where a lack of confidence stops you trying things or enjoying aspects of your life, then you need to give it a boost.

Older women in particular need to be confident. We are less likely to get complimented on our looks (we still will be, just less likely that's all). We are less likely to be included in conversations with younger people and we are less likely, in some situations, to be listened to at all, as if somehow our opinions are no longer valid. There are many older women who were confident when they were younger who suddenly lose it all, after just one or two of these experiences. But we have life experiences to impart to others, we have opinions, we like talking to people of all ages. So we need to speak out and to speak out on behalf of women of all ages. We are here to enjoy life so if you like dancing, dance and if you like chatting to new people, chat to new people and if you want to take up stand up comedy or rapping or naked snowboarding then have the confidence to give it a go.

The first thing you need is a determination that any lack of confidence you feel will NEVER stop you doing what you want to do deep down. The second thing you need to do is: CHANGE THE VOICE IN YOUR HEAD.

Is the voice in your head saying:-
'No one's going to listen to me…'
'I'm too old to….'
'AA Gill may have a point.'
'It's too late to do something different.'
'If only I was younger…'
'If only I looked different…'
'I wish I'd…'
'What if I fail?'
'Nothing will ever change.'

'It's a young man's world.'

Change all that to:-
'I'll give it a go.'
'It's never too late to….'
'I have so much experience to offer.'
'I deserve to…'
'I am interesting and have interesting viewpoints.'
'I feel comfortable as me.'
'I can, I will.'

This is all getting a bit American self help book. I'd better move on before I talk about your inner child and make reference to the fact that we're all on a journey. I realise though that you may be shouting at the book – 'It's all very well to say change the voice in your head, but how.'

I have to admit it isn't easy, especially if that negative voice has been there for some time. But it can be done. Firstly:
NOTICE YOUR NEGATIVE INNER VOICE

Sometimes it's such a habit, we don't even know we're doing it. Especially if the viewpoint that older women don't have much to contribute seems to be echoed in the society around us. But we know that's bullshit. So when you catch yourself with those unhelpful thoughts, shout STOP. (You can do a sort of internal shout if you're in the post office queue or in a meeting at work. Best to, really.) Then replace it with a positive one. Practice makes perfect. So stick with it. Now:
USE THE TIMES WHEN YOU ARE CONFIDENT.

There will be at least one aspect of your life where you DO feel comfortable in your own skin and confident with who you are. Maybe you're fine at work, or maybe you know you're a good cook. Maybe you're confident in your role as a parent or grandparent. It could be absolutely anything. And it will obviously be different for everyone. One woman's self esteem at cooking could be another's burnt sausage. Notice how you feel when you are doing the activity or are in the environment when you feel the most confident. Now focus on that feeling. Close your eyes and really feel it. Then next time you are in a situation where you feel less than confident – you know those times when you can't quite recall your own name and end up hiding in the toilets – then channel the confident you. Recall how you are in those confident situations and get yourself in that mindset. And then ask yourself:

WHAT'S THE WORST THAT CAN HAPPEN?

This is a really useful question. Obviously if you're hanging off the edge of a cliff then you might not want to focus on the worst case scenario. But usually the worst that can happen is that we make an arse of ourselves. So what? Think of situations where someone else has made themselves look like a little bit of a plonker. Chances are they laughed it off and so did everyone else. The worst that can happen, actually, is that we show how vulnerable we are. And showing your vulnerable, faulty self to others makes you very endearing. Do you really only like perfect people with shiny teeth who say exactly the right things and know how to hold the fish knives? Chances are those are exactly the sort of people you don't take to. Maybe the worst thing that can happen is you don't get that job, achieve that sporting ambition or team up with that George Clooney look-a-like. SO WHAT? You won't be any worse off than you were before. The same but with a bit of disappointment thrown in. And like all emotions, disappointment disappears in time. Quite a short period of time usually. Now ask yourself:

IS EVERY ONE ELSE REALLY CONFIDENT?

Look around you and clock everyone else's confidence levels. Do they seem way more confident than you? Really? Look again and note their body language. Are they fiddling with a paper clip, smoothing down their hair rather more often than necessary or maybe there's a man with a mop and bucket clearing up the pool of sweat at their feet. The truth is everyone can get nervous. Few people are confident in every situation. We tend to compare the inside of ourselves with the outside of others. And outer appearances can be deceptive. And while you're busy envying young people their natural confidence and exuberance, they are busy envying you. That's because young people assume older people are more confident on account of them having been around the block a few times.

It's possible that you were more confident when you were younger. Seeing older women being slated on Twitter and ignored on television doesn't do a great deal for our confidence. But you're the same person you used to be when you were younger, only more experienced. You deserve to be more confident, not less. If it's changes such as new technology which are knocking your confidence, then get up to speed. Remember there is no such thing as being too old. That's almost true. Not quite. I'm not likely to have another baby now. Or get acne.
GET A GOOD ROLE MODEL.

We know that nearly everyone has to work on their confidence every now and again. And that most people have one aspect of their life where they feel a little more confident. However, there are some older women out there who have a barrow load of confidence, both on the outside and on the inside. They're useful. They can be our role models. They are there for us to follow and to show the world that older women have an important role to play in our society. And if they can do it with confidence, so can we.

You can pick your own role model, whether it's Judi Dench or Maggie Smith, Oprah Winfrey or Hilary Clinton, Jenni Murray or Mary Beard (Take that AA). There are singers, actors, politicians, presenters, scientists, entrepreneurs who are women in the older category. So pick someone you admire and look at how they stand and hold themselves, how they talk, how they present themselves, their facial expressions. What makes them appear confident? Then close your eyes and STEP INTO THEIR SHOES.

You may be shouting out 'but they were good in their field from a young age, no wonder they're confident.' You may also be shouting out 'they wouldn't be able to achieve that if they'd started later in life.' Or even 'what right has AA Gill to have a go at any woman clearly more clever than him.' The last one is not really relevant. Well, it is. Very. But it was in a previous chapter. Still, can't mention it enough, really.

You may want to make your role model someone who achieved success in their field when they were a middle-aged or older woman. There are many women who started something new in later years and found they were very good at it. And women who had been trying to achieve something, whether getting a book published or singing to a large audience, for years and finally made it later in life. These role models made it in middle-age, disproving that voice in your head which is telling you it's too late. Here are a few examples.

Louise May Alcott was 37 when she published her first book. Not old enough? I agree. Laura Ingalls Wilder was 64 when she published Little House on the Prairie. And she was 76 when her last book (These Happy Golden Years) was published. Too long ago? There are many current examples such as Helen Dewitt who wrote her first novel, The Last Sumurai in her forties. And there are women who started later than that.

Kathryn Joosten, best known for her roles in Desperate Housewives and West Wing, didn't become an actor until her forties. Rene Russo (Lethal Weapon 3, Get Shorty) got her first role ages 43 and so on. Phyllis Diller started as a comedian in her late thirties and with the recent spurt in female comics, I am sure there will be those starting older than that. Anna Mary Robertson Moses (aka Grandma Moses) started painting at the age of 76. She worked for twenty five years, producing work which sold for over $10,000.

Mother Teresa was 40 when she left her old life behind to start the Missionaries of Charity organisation. She got the Nobel Peace Prize aged 69. And Susan Boyle was 48 when she made our jaws drop on Britain's Got Talent with her amazing rendition of 'I dreamed a dream'. And last but not least (well probably least, but not for my family) I was well into my fifties when I did my first performance poetry gig in 2013.

It can be done. There are women out there who had the confidence to get up and have a go at what they've always wanted to do. And succeeded. So they've paved the way for the rest of us.

However, I do have to ponder on the Susan Boyle factor. You must have seen clips of the moment this middle-aged woman came onto the X factor stage for her first audition. She did not look particularly glamorous, some even called her dowdy. The camera zoomed in onto Simon Cowell's face. He raised his eyes heavenwards as if to say 'this is going to be awful.' Yes, I know it's all staged and yes I know this was a clue that she was going to be brilliant. One line of the song in and we knew she was uber talented. The camera goes straight to Amanda Holden's face. Her jaw drops and she looks amazed. She is an actress, after all. The message was clear – we don't expect anything much from non-glamorous middle-aged women and when they actually can do something, it's a novelty. Fast forward a few weeks and the internet is alight with Susan Boyle jokes all focused on her looks. That's not a novelty. That's par for the course.

So yes, we do want a society that recognises the talents and achievements of all, despite their looks and their age and their gender. And this needs to be the norm so we do not have the Susan Boyle situation again. We want an older women, who may not be stylish, to come onto the X factor and we half expect she will be good. We want the press and the Twitterati to focus on their talent and refrain from misogynist, sexist comments. Yes, I dream a dream too.

I also want a world where I can easily list women who have made it later in life. I had to scrabble around a bit for this lot and have to admit, it would have been so much easier to list men who had made it later in life. And if Susan Boyle had been Stephen Boyle, then perhaps we would have been spared Simon's raised eyes and Amanda's jaw drop. Still, we have to start somewhere and there are older women who have succeeded IN ALL WALKS OF LIFE. Older women who go to university for the first time in their forties, older women who switch career in their forties and older women who get into politics in their forties. They are friends of mine. And you may have friends like that too. If you have a friend, colleague or acquaintance who can be your role model, then so much the better as this really will make it clear that it can be done. She will not be some celebrity who seems a world away from you, but a real woman you know. See how your role models have had the confidence to make a change, achieve whatever they've achieved and know that you can be like that too.

One of the most effective ways of learning golf, I am told, is to study the swings of the professionals and model your swing on theirs. I have no idea about golf but it sounds reasonable. And in the same way, study the confident woman you admire and do a bit of copying.

FAKE IT TO MAKE IT

It's all very well trying to channel Julie Andrews stepping off that bus and singing 'I have confidence in sunshine' when you know that you really only have confidence it's going to rain again. On you. Isn't modelling yourself on someone else really just pretending? Won't we just look confident on the outside while our internal organs are turning to bowls of wobbly jelly? Well yes, but with confidence you can start on the outside and work inwards. Here's why:

1. Try smiling. For three minutes. You don't have to have anything to smile about. Maybe you've just run over your cat or you've been passed over for promotion by a twelve year old. But smile anyway. After three minutes, how do you feel? Yes, much better. That's because a smile gets the endorphins going. So pretending to be happy works just as pretending to be confident works. They're sort of linked anyway. Confident people don't tend to walk into that board room in tears. Usually.

2. Change your posture. Shoulders back, stand tall, head up. Just like your mother used to tell you when you were thirteen and 'life is just so unfair.' How do you feel? Yes, it's as good as a smile - we should have all listened to our mothers. Do the confident posture and you will feel more confident.

3. Notice how other people respond to you when you are smiling and doing the confident posture. A confident posture is open – no closed arms across you as if the contents of your stomach might spill out onto the carpet, no head hanging down and to one side, like a broken nodding dog in the back of the car. And an open posture makes you more approachable. People will talk to you and all because you're pretending to be confident.

4. Remember something sad in your life and run it through your head. It can bring you to tears. Now make up something very sad happening. It can do the same. The unconscious mind doesn't know the difference between reality and fantasy. So fantasise about walking into that room and blowing them all away with your witty retorts and instant rapport. Now how do you feel? And you haven't even done

anything yet. Pretending to be confident has made you seem confident to others. And made you feel more confident too. It works – acting out confidence actually changes how you feel.

IMPOSTOR SYNDROME

I got quite excited when I found out about this, imagining women everywhere suddenly bursting into bad impersonations of Margaret Thatcher at inappropriate times. Or maybe pretending to be a close friend of Prince William to get into a posh private party. But it's neither of those. Impostor syndrome is very prevalent among professional women. It's where someone thinks they have got into their position by luck, that they really don't deserve to be there and that they WILL BE FOUND OUT at any moment. This affects both men and women but it appears that it affects women far more. The jury's out on this – early research back in 1978 when Abba were taking a chance on me and the Boomtown Rats were caught in a rat trap, suggested it was a woman thing. But more recent research isn't as clear. Stephen Brookfield, professor of St Thomas in Minneapolis St Paul knows all about it and he suggests that men get it too but that women are more likely to own up to it. Dr Valerie Young has written extensively on the subject too so you can take a look at some of her work. She too suggests men get it as well. But anecdotal evidence does lean towards it being far more prevalent in women.

Stephen Brookfield points out that a little bit of Impostor Syndrome is no bad thing and I agree. Having a syndrome generally implies too much of something that is quite normal in small amounts. It's normal to overindulge in chocolate occasionally but not normal to binge eat on a regular basis. A fear of new situations is normal but it's not normal to shut yourself away and not face the world, and so on. So it's normal to occasionally doubt whether you're up to the job but if it plagues your every thought and you're looking over your shoulder expecting someone to say – 'shouldn't you be cleaning the toilets,' then it's got out of hand. Brookfield points out that without a little touch of self doubt then you would be a megalomaniac who believes herself to be infallible.

I would go further and suggest it's often a disease of the older woman. It's been discovered that it is common among trail blazers – i.e. the first women in high political positions or in the board room or doing what was once considered to be a very male job such as engineering. And these trail blazers are now more likely to be older women. And there are also the women who see young bright sparks coming up behind them and begin to doubt whether they should be there. Once again, we tend to forget the extensive value of experience in this society.

You are in good company if you do have a touch of Impostor Syndrome – Tina Fey and Maya Angelou have both admitted to it among many other successful women. So, if you find yourself thinking 'they must have confused me with that intelligent women in the designer suit at the interview,' or 'I should be the waitress serving at this conference, not the delegate' or 'someone's going to spot me and send me back to the hospital where they'll analyse me for some sort of psychological disorder,' then you need to take action. You may even find yourself thinking you should never have had children or grandchildren put in your care or that your partner will suddenly discover you're a boring woman who looks like a creased up extra thick duvet when her clothes are off. It's all about lack of confidence and self esteem so all the advice in this chapter is particularly relevant to you. Further advice is:

1. Act confidentially but also have some humility – this way you can admit if you don't know something. Never feel you have to pretend you know it all. Why would you? (I know, we've

all done it.)

2. Most people with this syndrome tend to be perfectionists. Accept your faults. Accept your limitations if they genuinely are limitations. This may require some work - think of other people who have a few faults (we all do). I bet you accept their faults more readily than your own. Talk to yourself the way you would a best friend.

3. Use other people. You don't have to be able to know everything if you have people that do know at hand. Asking for help is not a weakness.

4. It's true – problems ARE opportunities.

5. Lose the self blame. Not everything can be your fault.

The new confident you is never going to think your achievements were some sort of fluke. You are not going to be affected by messages in our society which might suggest youth and beauty win every time. You will have the confidence to challenge discrimination against you and others. You will show that you offer value and experience where you work, where you live, where you socialise and to the world at large. You will lead the way for the next generation who don't know it yet, but will get older too. Wow. All this, just by making yourself smile and hold your head up when you walk in that room.

SEVEN: WHAT WE CAN TEACH THE NEXT GENERATION

I mainly ignored my mother. Yes, my mother who told me to smile, keep my shoulders back and my head up and face the world. I ignored that piece of advice from her and here I am putting it in a book to share with others. The truth is my mother and others of her generation did, from time to time, pass advice onto me and from time to time, I listened to it (but often didn't). And even more frequently, I've looked back and realised they probably were right about a number of things.

Having bigged up older women and ranted a lot about all the experience we have to offer the world, it goes to reason that we have a place in passing our knowledge and life's experience onto the next generation. But will they listen? If we look at who the role models are for the younger generation, you may be cheered to see that they just might. In 2012, a survey by the Girl Guides Association put Mum as the top role model for girls age eleven to twenty one. In 2011, a survey by Paramount Home Education found the top role model for girls was, you guessed it, their mum. And to save time, I'll summarise all the surveys asking girls who their top role model is. Mother. Yes, you. The one they called 'sad', the one they claimed didn't understand, the one they hated when you didn't allow them to stay out all night at an unknown location with dubious strangers. Underneath the teenage stroppiness, your daughter does actually look up to you. They may be in their twenties before they fully realise this and eventually admit it but you are a role model, even if at times you feel like a cross between a prison officer and a Downton Abbey servant. Only without the big house and the silver.

Usefully for this book, my daughters are in their twenties and I was able to ask them how I had influenced them. I asked them to be honest (knowing I could edit their comments if necessary) but the results were pretty cheering. It seems I have, over the years, passed on some of my experience to them and that it has influenced how they are living their lives. The only bit I edited out was both my daughters' remarks about my lack of sewing prowess. But then maybe I've passed my wit and humour onto them. If you can call sarcasm humour.

Eldest daughter, Emma, declares 'I have adopted some of your philosophy and outlook on life. I often find myself quoting you on this – for example, the other day I advised a friend about how we all have different journeys and you should focus on your own path rather than comparing your own life to others. I have also learned the value of hard work, determination and never giving up. I have learned an appreciation of books and poetry and the value of lifelong learning. I have learned resilience and the ability to take on whatever life throws at me. And I have learnt to make a good béchamel sauce.'

My younger daughter, Jessica, sent me a list. You will know by now that I'm rather partial to a list so there's a bit of rubbing off spotted before I've even read it. Included in her 30 point list, was 'If you're stuck on something, go for a walk,' 'Do something towards your dream each day,' 'You get out of life what you put into it,' and 'listen to Kate Bush'. I was particularly pleased that feminism was top of the things I have passed on to her. At the end she wrote 'you taught me the morals and values by which I try to live my life.'

So there we have it. Job done. Except their father played quite a part in passing on stuff too (not the béchamel sauce but he does all the sewing in our house). It seems I have passed down a mixture of knowledge (the sauce) and experience (resilience) personality (determined) and passion (poetry and books). I asked the same question of a young woman in her twenties I used to work with and I had a similar response – hard work and determination were mentioned as well as my experience and knowledge in the job. So, we do have positive things to pass down to the next generation, there's no doubt. It seems the young do see the value in experience and accumulated knowledge so it's surely our duty to mix in with the next generation, talk together, work together, socialise together, share common interests together. A good argument against having under twenty five playwriting groups or over sixties swimming clubs or thirty something book groups (yes, there is one!)

This is all very positive. Middle-aged women pass down all their knowledge, experience and wisdom. We know exactly how to live our lives, so we show the next generation down and we, well, explain it all to them. Like a sort of driving instructor for life. Except even driving instructors have crashes or break the speed limit. So here's the next question – can the next generation learn from our mistakes?

There was some interesting research done in Bristol in 2010 led by Dr Paul Howard-Jones and Dr Rafel Bogacz. They asked volunteers to play a computer game against an artificial opponent and looked at their brain scans. It transpired that the players learnt from their own successes but had very little reaction to the artificial opponent's win. But when the computer made mistakes and failed, brain activity jumped up. However, anecdotal advice seems mixed. For example, it has been shown if you were smacked as a child, you are more likely to smack your own children. And yet, I made a conscious decision to try and not smack my children because I have bad memories of being hit for no reason. I like to think I at least attempted to learn from my parents' mistakes. I'm not the best cook in the world, but it seems my daughters were determined to learn from my burnt offerings and turned themselves into far better cooks than I am. But a friend of mine reports that her daughter has 'followed in her footsteps' and drinks, smokes and swears exactly like she does. Though despite these 'faults', I have to say both this mother and her daughter are the kindest, most generous people I know.

It seems to me, that the younger generation will learn from us when they want to learn from us, taking in our good and bad bits of role modelling and making what they can of it all. In the early years, we are just role models and our daughters will mimic us without question. Look at the five year old putting on high heels and smearing lipstick round her mouth so she can be just like Mummy. This is the age when they unconsciously take in the things we don't want to model. Like smoking. In the teenage years, they will then try and break away and are likely to go out of their way to be as unlike us as possible. But that early modelling has a deep rooted effect. So even if they don't want to smoke like us, it's already there in the unconscious mind. As is the fact that they saw us reading. Taking them to pantomimes and children's plays when they are young is far more likely to install an interest in theatre than suddenly taking them to Macbeth at thirteen.

So we have influenced our daughters and other young people we've known as they've grown up. But should we also be influencing them in a way which will prepare them for being middle-aged themselves? Why not? Maybe the next generation will be more prepared for middle-ageddom. And maybe they can have the confidence we sometimes lack. If we can pave the way to ensure there is less discrimination against older women, then they can thank us as we all thank the suffragettes and those seventies feminists who achieved new equality laws. If my own mother showed me that being middle-aged meant sitting in dowdy clothes, slowly disintegrating into a pile of useless bones and lost dreams, then we can show our daughters it's the age of bungee jumping, karaoke and changing the world. We can show them that life just gets better and better, which it has the potential of doing. We can show them that you never stop learning, you never stop living and you never stop to regret. Because that's how it should be. That's how it can be.

Why do we fear getting older? Obviously, we're not too keen on the getting closer to death bit. But we're also not too keen on the losing our vitality bit. We're not keen on losing our worth in society as our children fly the nest and we face retirement with its years of gardening, creaky bones and sitting in a conservatory wondering where the years went. Why do we fear that? Because we can think of our own parents, aunts and uncles, friends and neighbours who are doing just that. But these days, we can also think of older people working until they want to give up (not to a specific age), heading off to yoga, the gym or beach volley ball and taking up new activities and even new jobs.

I was the last to leave home and I remember my mother crying. She felt she had lost an important role and that she was no longer needed as a mother (I did my bit to help by continuing to ask for bail outs when I went overdrawn. Hope that helped). But some women see it as a positive time. Time for them to do things for themselves for a change. The experience of my mother's loss when we all left impacted on my own fear of my daughters leaving home. When my mother finally gave up work, she took to a lot of polishing and phoning me up rather more often than was necessary. I grew up with a rather negative view of getting older. It seemed to mean losing your identity. But in reality it can mean the opposite. Many women really find themselves in middle-age and beyond. No longer thought of as someone's mother and partner, perhaps financially a little more stable, they can start new things in their life.

It's not just important for ourselves that we continue to grow and take risks, it's important for the generation below. We are their role models, whether we like it or not. Show them the joys of getting older. Demonstrate that life can go on getting more exciting and more challenging. Fight against ageism and sexism to pave the way for them. And for goodness sake, spend time with younger people. They can't learn from you or benefit from your experience if you sit on your own in your dressing gown eating chips or have never moved on from the two old school friends you still insist on spending every weekend with. Have friends of all ages, spend time with your daughters and nieces, don't automatically head for the table in the works canteen which looks like a meeting for the menopausal. And while the young are busy benefitting from your experience, you'll be learning from them too.

One of the contestant's from The Great British Bake Off, seventeen year old Martha Collison, described how she felt about being on a programme where all the other contestants were much older than her. She told us how she felt nervous and uncomfortable about it. But she admits she need not have been because these older bakers BECAME LIFELONG FRIENDS. We are conditioned to think our friends must be the same age as us but friends of different ages can learn from each other and break down the generation barriers which we have somehow built. I bet Martha benefitted from some of the life experience of the older women on the programme. And I bet they fed off her youthful enthusiasm and vitality.

But what is this experience we're talking about? I just took a break to listen to the wonderful Woman's Hour on Radio 4. Jane Garvey (age 49) was interviewing one of their power listers, Martha Lane Fox (age 40). They began to discuss an accident Martha had been involved in and Jane pointed out that there hadn't been a single woman she had interviewed as part of this power list, where something dramatic like this hadn't happened. And that's partly what the experience of the older woman is. You simply don't get to age forty or fifty without something happening to you. No one, I repeat no one, lives some sort of charmed life where everything runs smoothly, there are no problems and life turns out exactly as we planned and expected. We might meet women where that seems to be the case, but dig just a little bit beneath the surface and you'll find problems and events from the past which were, at best, challenging.

The chances are you'll have been through a divorce, death of someone close to you, miscarriage, loss of a job, been a victim of crime, made some blundering great mistake, made a disastrous choice or been through a period of poor health. You'll be lucky if only one of those things have happened (and extremely unlucky if they all have.) That's life and guess what? You're still here. A little bruised by life's events maybe but still here to tell the tale. And tell the tale you must. I don't mean spew out the details of your divorce to a complete stranger at the bus stop or paste up post op photos on Facebook. But when you meet someone younger going through something that you've been through, then tell them about you. Not in great detail but enough for them to think – hey, she went through this AND SHE SURVIVED.

It's also our duty to dispel a few myths about growing a little older. You will have discovered by now that hitting forty does not mean you have turned into an alien from another planet. You will also have discovered that you don't really feel any different to when you were twenty five. And there are plenty of other unfounded stories which are believed by young and old alike. Let's look at the ten myths of ageing.

MYTH NUMBER ONE:
Brains don't work very well any more.
WRONG. Although cells die off as we get older, new ones can grow. German researcher, Janina Boyke et al looked at brain scans of sixty year olds after they'd been taught to juggle. The scans showed growth in the grey matter that processes complex visual information. And if you don't fancy juggling as a new career, you can learn a new language or an instrument or whatever. Alongside younger people. And hold your own. When

I recently had to learn some poetry for performance, I was convinced I would struggle and felt overawed by my actress daughter, Jessica, who learns her lines in seconds. BUT I GOT THE HANG OF IT. And I like to think I may have grown a few neurons along the way.

MYTH NUMBER TWO:
You get more and more boring as you age.
WRONG. There are loads of examples of older women doing amazing and sometimes crazy things. Yo to 93 year old Tao Porchon-Lynch who has a dance partner of 23 and wins ballroom dancing competitions across America (when she's not teaching yoga classes). Well done to all the over fifty year old runners in the 2013 London Marathon. Especially the ones in fancy dress. And especially 83 year old, Iva Barr. Good fun from forty year old Viv Groskop who took up stand up and wrote a book about it. And big respect to fifty year old Jenny from Essex who offers free hugs at railways stations. And gets a very good response.

MYTH NUMBER THREE:
You get more miserable.
A sweeping generalisation. Obviously some people get more miserable but research suggests the opposite is more likely. A study in 2004 by Laura Carstensen from Stanford University asked people to look at cheerful, distressing and neutral pictures. The brains of the younger group (aged 18-29) were activated equally by both the cheerful and the distressing pictures. The older group (70-90) reacted more to the positive pictures. So there you are – we gradually focus on the positive as we get older. A 2007 study published in the Journal of Gerontology asked people to solve hypothetical social problems. It concluded that as you get older, you are more socially intelligent and so less likely to get into arguments. The argumentative, grumpy old git is a

myth then.

MYTH NUMBER FOUR:
Bodies and minds slowly disintegrate.
We've dealt with the brain bit in Myth Number One, but I'm mentioning it here as, although our bodies don't get any younger, you can do an awful lot to prevent bones shrinking, muscles withering and your mind slowing up. Exercise. If you keep moving, your brain as well as your body keeps 'young.' So no, you don't have to slow down mentally or physically. Always best to find the sort of exercise you enjoy as you are more likely to keep it up.

MYTH NUMBER FIVE:
You get stuck in a rut.
Again, not if you don't want to. Research has shown that older people adapt to new experiences and places more easily because they have a wealth of experience to tap into. So do something you've never done before. Now.

MYTH NUMBER SIX:
We stop learning.
NO, NO, NO. Look at myth number one – our brains can still expand, we can keep learning new things right till the end. And you will whether you want to or not. For example, it has been shown that our vocabulary carries on expanding until well into old age. Just think of all the new technological terms you now use without thinking every time you log onto a computer.

MYTH NUMBER SEVEN:
We spend all our time watching Countdown.
Actually, we prioritise far better as we get older. It's thought that's because we become increasingly aware that our time here is

limited. Young people seem to have very little concept of the future, let alone death. The middle-aged may have lost one or both parents and are suddenly made aware that it's them next. They are more likely to have lost friends and relatives. And with that increased awareness of life being far from endless, we don't want to waste any time and so get a stronger sense of what's important. That doesn't mean none of you think watching Countdown's a good use of your time, some of you may love it, but it does mean you are more likely to have made a definite CHOICE to watch it rather than just finding yourself slumped in front of it.

MYTH NUMBER EIGHT:
We want to spend the inheritance.

A study by Sumit Agarwi, an economist at the Federal Reserve Bank of Chicago, found older people made better decisions about money and the peak for this was in our early fifties. This may not be much of a myth to be honest. We seem to have a younger generation very comfortable living their lives in debt. It probably all begins with student loans but I can't help thinking it was easier when we used to hold real money in our hands rather than an oblong of plastic. Perhaps this is something important we can pass down to the next generation – living within your means. And I would like to see money awareness taught in schools. In the mean time, I have told my daughter to refuse credit cards and overdraft facilities until she is earning more. I have even suggested she takes her money out for the week in cash so she can actually see how much she's got. Or maybe write down everything she spends. I mention this as an example of how in some situations, trying to pass on the benefit of our experience simply doesn't work. This daughter remains hopeless with money.

MYTH NUMBER NINE:

We get pickier.

Actually, research suggests the opposite, that we are more able to see the bigger picture. A 2005 study carried by Allison Sekuter in the Mcmaster University of Canada asked people to point out shapes on the screen. To cut a complicated piece of research short, the older age groups were better with bigger shapes where there was more contrast and the younger candidates were better with small grey shapes. No, I didn't quite understand the task either. But the conclusion is that young brains are better at focusing on details but to the exclusion of their surroundings. It would suggest that with more years of experience, we are able to look at a situation and immediately get the overall meaning of what is happening – the bigger picture. I also think us older women use our intuition more effectively to sum up situations and get a grasp of what we are looking at. Intuition partly involves using previous experience to draw unconscious conclusions about people, places and events. And we have more experience than the younger generation. Stands to reason that we have a more finely tuned intuition.

MYTH NUMBER TEN:

You stop having sex at about forty.

Each generation thinks they invented sex. No. And you can go on having it into your eighties and nineties. Shirley Conran, in her eighties, admits to being sexually active and this is not unusual. Charlie Chaplin, among others, fathered a child in his nineties. And he didn't find it under a gooseberry bush next to a stork. And yes, your parents and grandparents have sex. And yes, they like it too. Young people didn't invent it any more than the older generation did. It started back in the beginning of time. And it hasn't changed that much.

If you can help dispel some of the myths then younger people won't see us as some other species who are likely to forget their own name at any minute, will launch into some dull ramble about the good old days and only really want a comfy chair and a nice cup of tea of an evening. When they see us at our liveliest, most creative and most fun then there is more likelihood of some intergenerational activities, friendships and mutual support.

It has been said many times in recent years that the youth are information rich and knowledge poor. It never ceases to amaze me how easy it is to get information. The Google generation have never had to scour libraries, use weighty encyclopaedias, troll through the yellow pages to find experts or ask a man down the pub who might know a man who knows a woman who can help. I wrote some parenting books in the pre-internet era. I had worked with children and had a certain amount of expertise myself. But I also wanted to consult other experts and look at the research. I scoured the shelves of the local university library, I wrote letters (yes, letters and on paper) and asked questions of experts. I found people in directories and telephoned them. And they answered me on a phone that was attached to the wall as they sat at their desks, piled high with paper. It was hard work, accumulating that extra knowledge about child development and parenting. But oh how much easier it would be to write those books now. How relatively simple it is to look up research and expert opinions for this book. But needless to say, there is more information out there than I need. Now, the work is not in finding the information but in knowing what to do with it. And that is what we mean by information rich, knowledge poor.

The younger generation have always had information at their fingertips. It comes in short bites – a blog rather than an essay, a column rather than a feature, lists rather than analysis. It's an age of instant gratification. We want an answer to that question and we want it now. And we can get it now. Without really having to think first. It was nearly thirty years ago that a similar expression was coined by psychologist and computer scientist, Herbert Simon – information rich and attention poor. Again, this is about wanting it instantly and in bite size chunks. Maybe the information we have at the press of a key board lacks depth and maybe, to some degree, the thinking is done for us. And we don't have to remember anything anymore. We can just look it up again. On our phones. Without having to go anywhere near a library.

How does this fit in with our quest to 'teach' the younger generation? I'm certainly not suggesting that we throw away our daughters' lap tops and buy them a set of encyclopaedias and a library card for Christmas, saying – here you go, now you can really learn some research skills. But we can open up discussions in an intergenerational situation. The advantages of digital information are enormous, but it is enhanced by talking about this new information. Information becomes knowledge once we have thought about it, analysed it, made connections to information we have already acquired and remembered it. And we can help by being part of the analysis through discussion and debate.

Which brings me to word of mouth. Not all information and knowledge is acquired via a computer, and there is a still a place, in fact a NEED, to pass on information, knowledge and tradition orally. We can keep that oral tradition alive without losing the advantages of technology. I still remember things my mother taught me, I still remember stories she told me, I still recall the little family traditions we had from what we did at Christmas to the little jokes we had about each other which became ingrained in the culture of my family.

I recently attended a workshop with the story teller Louise Coigley and it was fascinating. She told, and then we told, stories which had been passed down from generation to generation in a huge variety of cultures across the world. Many of these started by being passed down orally long before they were written down. The fairy tales written by the brothers Grimm were simply traditional folk tales which had been passed down by word of mouth which they then adapted and wrote down. I tell my children stories of my childhood and of my mother's childhood which she told me. I can imagine some of these family stories of our lives will be passed down to another generation. And I remember them. I can tell you all about my Grandmother playing tennis at Wimbledon or the time my Uncle ran away from the farm because he'd hit his father and how my mother used to walk miles to school. And my children know of these things too. They are not written down but we know them. We understand what the incidences and events meant to the people involved because this is more than information, it's knowledge acquired from someone else's experience. So we can help the next generation turn all that information into knowledge by talking about what it all means to us.

The suggestion posed by this chapter title is that we have something to teach the next generation just as we learnt from our mothers. It's clear that no amount of technology can take the place of direct learning from others. Whether it's by listening to their stories, gaining insight from their experience or looking at someone we admire and aspire to be like as a model for ourselves. A list is long overdue.

We can teach the next generation:

1. Tradition. Pass down family traditions and family stories.
2. Experience. Share your experiences good and bad. Your children (and other younger people in your life) will inevitably have to make their own mistakes but they will eventually draw on the benefit of your life's successes and

failures.

3. Attributes we have gained with time. We tend to be calmer and more measured. We tend to see the bigger picture. Believe it or not we worry less.

4. The myths of growing older. You can help dispel the myths we have discussed by being that energetic, up-for-anything, feisty woman who is not so very different from the younger you. No pressure though - feeling a bit drowsy after lunch is the middle-age equivalent of teenagers unable to leave their beds in the morning.

5. That we are not a separate species. We are all women and need to share and mix and collaborate.

6. We also desperately need to teach our daughters about sexism and what we should NEVER put up with. They need to get some confidence and self respect from somewhere as there are too many young girls being cajoled into taking part in things they are not comfortable with. We need frank and open discussion with them about all things sexual. From pre-teenager upwards. But we need to accept that it is peer support which can also play a big part in making changes so encourage her to talk to friends. Peer support in other areas of concern, such as bullying, has been the most effective, so accept we are only a small part of the solution, but a part nonetheless.

7. We must also teach our sons about respect and make sure they are aware that violent sex or sex which demeans women is NOT the norm. Again, you need frank and open on going discussions about this, however uncomfortable.

8. We might as well teach them a bit about ageism too, while we're about it.

Mixing up the generations is something I'm very keen on. I enjoy the company of people younger than myself and people much older. My daughters and their friends keep me young, very much older women help me understand life, children teach me more than anyone. Which brings me to a very important point. Learning is a two way street. While we're busy trying to pass on the wisdom of our experience to the next generation, they have a thing or two to teach us as well.

EIGHT: WHAT THE NEXT GENERATION CAN TEACH US

First of all, I promise that I will endeavour to get through this chapter without mentioning the phrase – Inner Child. Although I may mention the child-like aspects of ourselves. I just won't call it inner child, that's all.

Everyone I asked about this gave one answer immediately – technology. Then they went on to consider other things. But let's just deal with the five-year-old-computer-expert situation first. There's no need to go on about how quickly technology has changed. I remember having an electric typewriter and thinking I was ahead of the game. And it really wasn't that long ago when you think about it. Obviously, a generation who grew up eating microchips for breakfast are going to be very speedy at keeping up with the newest technological invention or fad. A lot of older people can be very resistant and often defensive. This can be a fear of change, an urge to cling on to the old or a fear that they will be slow to learn and will therefore be shown up in some way. But IT IS ESSENTIAL TO BE UP TO SPEED WITH TECHNOLOGY TO SURVIVE.

Soon all banking will be on line, it is much cheaper to pay bills on line and so on. Yes, I too mourn the loss of writing letters. But you can do both e mails and letters. You can meet friends for coffee and message them on Facebook. You can write your opinions and complaints to the local paper and twitter it all. You can play vinyl or stick it in your ears. But if you cling to the old exclusively, you will MISS OUT.

I admit to being a step behind my daughters on all things technical. But they have helped me to keep up to speed. I used to work in a department where I noticed the younger members of staff were a little quicker on the computer systems than I was. They were delighted to help. They loved knowing more than me.

Learning from the young is a win-win situation. Of course, it's a bit of a stereotype – older people being slow at technology, as there are also younger people who don't like aspects of technology. But stereotypes, while being very annoying for those who don't fit in with it, are based on a tendency. And there has been a tendency for older people to be less au fait with all things computerised. However, this is changing. It needs to, so don't be the one left behind. If you really are far from being up to speed, grab someone who knows what you need to know or sign up for a course. So that's technology dealt with very simply - keep up.

I find the next generation lacking (mostly) in cynicism, they are nearly always at the forefront of any campaign you care to mention with their passion bursting through. They demonstrate to us that we have to keep fighting for what we believe in. They have not yet had time to get themselves in a rut and so can show us how to keep moving forward. I once quoted that famous phrase 'give me the strength to accept the things I cannot change' to a twenty something who firmly told me that anything can be changed. She may not be technically correct but I admire her doggedness and have never used that tired old phrase since. I find the next generation to be largely full of hope, to have strong imaginations and most of all, they nearly all know how to have fun.

Yes, people of all ages can have fun so why do I get a strong sense that it comes more easily to the younger generation? This is where I am tempted to talk about your inner child, but the truth is that we all have to remind ourselves that having fun is the best way of relaxing and increasing our happiness quota. I recently went to a concert in Hyde Park and was envious of the young people rushing to the front, dancing, singing and laughing as if there was no tomorrow. I realised I was feeling inhibited where they most certainly weren't so I let go of my inhibitions and joined in. I can't recommend this strongly enough.

I admit to a tendency of saying 'the old songs are the best.' Then I met a couple of teenagers who loved current music but also listened to the Beatles and Stones, James Taylor and Joni Mitchell. They had the best of both worlds and that is exactly what we can do. Enjoy the old and bring on the new. Younger people seem to be rather better at this than I am. But I'm working on it.

I've used the term young people to mean young adults. But it's been said by many a guru that we can learn from children, so let's consider them further. Paulo Coelho, one of those aforementioned gurus, said 'a child can teach an adult three things – to be happy for no reason, to always be busy with something and to know how to demand with all his might that which he desires.'

Being happy for no reason and being busy are linked, in my mind, and it all comes down to mindfulness. Children are busy in a different way from our incessant busyness. We're drowning in our efforts to juggle work, family life, and at least five worries which are constantly spinning round in our mind. We're busy but we're not necessarily focused. Children have the advantage of not having to worry about paying bills or getting to a meeting on time but we can still learn from what to me seems to be a natural mindfulness. When you watch a child play you will see joy in the moment. You will often see focus on the game. When you see a little girl pretending to be a squirrel she really is a squirrel. She's not thinking – I'll be a squirrel until half past four and then I'll read a book. She's not thinking of the next thing, she's too busy being a squirrel. And she's being happy in that moment, whatever else is going on in her life.

Quite simply, children rarely worry about tomorrow, they express themselves freely, they are often fearless, and they live their life fully. I recommend spending time with children – this isn't always easy if your children are grown up and you haven't become a grandparent. So visit friends with children and if you have time, volunteer to hear them read in your local primary. You will find that their natural joy and mindfulness will rub off.

Obviously not all children have a happy, carefree childhood with endless parental love and lots of skipping through daisies. But there is some truth in the saying – children are very resilient. I am not dismissing childhood problems and anxieties, but nevertheless, I have observed children from very stressful backgrounds, putting all that behind them as soon as they are faced with a room full of toys and time to get down and really play. That's simply because play is therapeutic. All that mindfulness you get with play blocks out everything else. At least for a while.

Why don't adults play? We do, of course. We play sport, we have hobbies and we sing and dance. Adult play tends to be structured and purposeful. It tends to have rules and time limits and it tends to be led by other adults. It is, of course, really important to have our leisure time and to be creative. But can we also play like children play – with fewer limitations and no expectations for an outcome of any sort? Have you ever walked past the play park and felt an urge to get on that swing or slide? Most of us have. We all have a need for some pointless fun play. I'm not suggesting you turf a six year old off the swing and stay on it for an hour, not letting anyone else have a turn. However, do hang a block of wood off a tree in your garden or somewhere in some local woods and go ahead and swing.

The ideas for real, pointless, fun play are endless. Splash in the puddles in your wellies, pretend to be Adele when you sing in the shower, hold a fancy dress party where everyone has to act out their character for the duration of the party, throw snowballs or handfuls of autumn leaves at your partner, build sandcastles, blow bubbles, skip, get out some felt pens and doodle. And pretend to be a squirrel. Pretending is really underrated and yet we can all do it. My twenty something daughter pretended to be a Victorian woman fallen from grace who had contracted TB when she had a cold recently. And we all pretend to be the winner of X factor when singing in the shower (or is that just me?) There's an inner child in all of us. There, I couldn't avoid it in the end. But yes, even if it sounds like a 1970s self help book, GET IN TOUCH WITH YOUR INNER CHILD. And if being with children and watching children helps you achieve this, then do just that.

It seems to me that a key part of making the most of being an older woman is to mix with other generations so we can learn off each other and push down any boundaries between us. There are even organisations to promote this principle. Take your daughters to work schemes are popular in Canada and the USA, though haven't really caught on here yet. And there are several programmes across the country linking school children with retired people. I'd like to mix it up even more so that it isn't just the very young and the very old who are being bought together, but that we live in a country where all ages have a good time and learn from each other. We don't necessarily need schemes for this or take your daughter to work days and the like, but they can help kick start this.

So, we all learn from each other and we all live happily ever after. Certainly, more understanding of the middle-aged and older woman by other sections of society will help. But we still have to be mindful of the fact that there is discrimination against women and older people. Put the two together and we have a bit of a battle on our hands. Because we mustn't accept ageism and sexism as a way of life. We must do all we can to move towards total equality. Every individual must challenge any inequality they come up against. Time to be an adult again.

NINE: CHALLENGING AGEISM AND SEXISM

We have already discussed the legal aspects of discrimination. Every woman needs to be aware of this. It is surprising how many older women just accept that they are likely to be replaced at work by someone younger, that it's fine for a colleague to make tasteless jokes about her age, that it's acceptable to see older male presenters while their female counterparts disappear. It's as if it's been in our culture so long, we stop noticing it. But then as soon as you start talking about it, even those apparently accepting women and men realise that there's a problem. The penny drops. At least I hope it does.

Then there are the perfectly legal aspects of life we sense are no longer acceptable in a society which aims to be equal and non-discriminatory. Things like page three models or women in business expected to go to strip joints to entertain clients, or older women being patronised. Not acceptable.

Just in case there are any women or men reading this who want to say 'calm down, dear' to me or try and persuade me that there's nothing left to fight for, let's have some lists to show why we still need feminism and why we still need to fight ageism.

20 REASONS WE STILL NEED FEMINISM

1. Not enough girls are achieving their potential. (Only one in ten engineers is a woman, one in five architects is a woman and so on.)
2. Women are still not equally represented in many important areas of life such as parliament and in the boardroom.
3. Two women a week are killed by a partner or former partner in the UK.
4. 70% of people in the world living in poverty are women.
5. Calling someone a girl is considered to be an insult.

6. One woman gets raped every nine minutes. We are NOT asking for it.
7. FGM
8. Forced marriages and child brides.
9. Total ban on abortion in some societies.
10. Honour killings.
11. Women's sports are not televised to the same extent as men's.
12. Forced prostitution.
13. Women are portrayed in limited roles in advertisements.
14. Some comedians still think telling tasteless and unfunny rape jokes is a good idea.
15. Killing female babies or rating girls lower than boys still exists in some societies.
16. Women have a one in four chance of being a victim of domestic abuse.
17. Women enjoying a night out are called 'laddish'.
18. We should apparently be flattered when a group of men whistle or shout out very personal comments about our appearance.
19. Women of all ages are judged by how they look to a far greater extent than men.
20. We still earn less than men.

20 REASONS WHY WE NEED TO FIGHT AGEISM

1. Older women are given a clear message by the media to look younger.
2. Grey hair is considered to be shameful by some (and it only applies to women).
3. Older women are not represented on television enough.
4. Older people are often passed by for promotion despite laws.
5. Older people find it harder to get jobs, purely because of their age.

6. It is supposed to be funny to call an older woman an 'old dear' or 'old duck.'
7. Older and middle-aged people are stereotyped in advertisements. Or even on signposts - look at the one for elderly crossing the road. Not all old people have a stick and are bent over nearly double!
8. People are called 'middle-aged' as an insult.
9. It is assumed anyone over fifty has little energy.
10. It is assumed anyone over fifty is slow – physically and mentally.
11. Middle-aged women rarely appear on magazine covers.
12. When they do, they are airbrushed out of reality.
13. The menopause is looked on as a disease that stops women functioning.
14. It is assumed that the middle-aged had it too good when they were younger and need to pay for it now.
15. Older people do not feel they are respected for their experience.
16. AA Gill vs. Mary Beard is not an isolated case.
17. Some women feel the need to lie about their age.
18. We are asked our date of birth in situations where it is really not relevant.
19. Middle-aged women consistently report that they feel invisible.
20. There is ageism in insurance – car and medical in particular.

The first thing you will notice about these lists is that perhaps the most serious items are on the feminism list. There is certainly some urgency and necessity in tackling FGM and domestic violence and these need to be top of every agenda we have. But that's not to dismiss lives ruined by ageism where women suffer from depression triggered by ridiculous expectations on appearance or where women are forced out of work by ageist managers. It's all important and we owe it to ourselves and the next generation NEVER TO ACCEPT any amount of ageism or sexism.

When we are trying to fight for any change in attitude, there will be resistance, of course. Not everyone sees ageism or sexism as a problem and we can find ourselves talking to brick walls of men (and sometimes women) who just don't get it. Or maybe they just don't want to. But we have to keep trying. Look at the recent abuse on Twitter of certain feminists – there was no way they should give up on Twitter or their cause or else what was the point in fighting for it at all? So, let's start with the first thing we need to do, which is:-

MAKE EVERYONE AWARE

1. Remember that not everyone becomes engrossed with articles about feminist attitudes. There are still those who think that feminism has reached its objectives and we can all calm down. So have facts and figures at your finger tips about the ongoing issues from FGM to magazine images to the pay gap. Know about women forced out of presenting on television and be aware of the number of women who have illegally been made to retire early. Get googling. Precise knowledge is better than a vague rant.

2. But don't become a feminist bore. Other feminists won't get bored and will talk all day, but there's no point preaching to the converted. It would be like a double glazing salesman coming round to talk about how wonderful your existing double glazing is. Entertain your friends and colleagues with your knowledge. Yes, entertain. This does not necessarily mean quoting equality laws while juggling milk bottles. Find your own way of drawing your audience in. Humour does work, by the way.

3. When it comes to your own personal grievances, make the important people in your life aware. No good moaning to your best mate that Barry from accounts insists on calling you an old fossil of a dinosaur, tell Barry. Gently explain why you don't like it and if he tells you that you have no sense of humour, knee him in the testicles. No, delete that last thought. Ask Barry to come with you to discuss it with the manager. And if he won't come with you, then go on your own. See, it's like any conflict in a war zone – best to try the gently, gently negotiating first before getting the big guns out (or your knee).

4. Don't forget the power of the crowd. Causes are much harder to fight on your own. This might mean joining a feminist group, joining on line awareness campaigns and putting your name to causes you believe in. On a more local level, it might mean joining forces with other older women in your office or work place to ensure everyone gets it. Sometimes colleagues are just completely unaware of what's going on. Fill them in with what they need to know.

5. Write letters and features for your local press or on line magazines pointing out difficulties older women face. I would suggest writing a book but hey, just recommend this one.

DON'T ACCEPT THE STATUS QUO

1. Once everyone is aware of the difficulties, don't accept anything less than respect and equality. Just because something's been done for years, doesn't always mean it's right or fair. There was once a time when it was perfectly acceptable for women to get paid less than men FOR EXACTLY THE SAME JOB. There are now laws against this and pretty well the whole of society thinks equal pay laws are

absolutely right and proper. Of course, now inequality in pay is more subtle and less obvious but it's still not fair. So don't accept that traditionally female jobs such as speech therapists or pre-school teachers should be paid less than similar or equitable jobs more often done by men. And don't accept that women can not so readily progress up the pay ladder. And never accept that bearing children should impede your career.

2. When laws change, it takes a while for attitudes to follow sometimes. You no longer have to retire at a set age but if you are fit and able, can carry on. Good. But unfortunately there are some who have a negative view of older people and are not keen on them staying in a job they are good at. The law is on your side. So help change attitudes in your work place as well.

3. Attitudes to age are gradually changing. They say fifty is the new forty, sixty is the new fifty and so on. Soon eighty will be the new teenager - keep pushing those boundaries.

4. You really don't have to wear a plastic hat in the rain just because you've turned sixty. You don't have to clean the oven just because you've got ovaries. You can date someone from One Direction when you're forty. Challenge age and gender stereotypes. Always.

5. Equally, don't accept that you have to be younger than your years. If you want a pint of Ovaltine, have one. If you are in your sixties and WANT to retire, retire.

TAKE ACTION

1. You've decided something is unacceptable, even if it's part of a culture. You've alerted everyone involved. But nothing changes. So take action. Start a local or national campaign or put your name to a local or national campaign.

2. If you are fighting a specific cause personal to you, such as being discriminated against at work, then get a team on your side. This might include colleagues, the citizen's advice bureau, a lawyer, your union, your MP or an online help forum.

3. Gather together all the evidence you need. Records of specific incidents of discrimination, dates and witnesses. Get details of laws and work policies together and make a whinge into a proper campaign.

4. Go on line and see if you can contact others who have been discriminated against because of their age, sex or both. Don't re-invent the wheel, learn from those who have gone before you.

5. Don't leave others to take action. For bad to succeed, the good only have to do nothing.

I want to go back to the point about arming yourself with facts and figures to support your arguments. I suggest you are selective about your information. Pick the statistics which really drive your point home and don't be tempted to bombard a stranger at the bus stop with everything you know about age and sex discrimination. There's enough shocking statistics out there for a bus journey from John O'Groats to Lands End and the chances are your bus journey isn't going to be that long. And if it is, the chances are your 'victim' will hop off the bus long before you've even got out of the town. The trouble is we're living in a time of information overload. A weekly edition of the New York Times contains more information than a woman in the 17th Century would have got in a lifetime! And we now consume more than three times as much information as people did in the sixties. It's a bit like offering me a box of chocolates straight after I'd indulged in a huge three course meal. Even I wouldn't be able to polish off the whole box so I'll pick the strawberry cream and the nutty one and leave the rest. So we have to decide which information we want to pay attention to and which we will either ignore or leave for another day. And if you're trying to get someone on your side about issues, they will be selective too. So pick the facts and stats you really need.

You could argue that we're also suffering an overload of groups and websites and twitterites and campaigns all pretty much shouting for the same thing. I don't really have a problem with that. I believe we need local campaigns, national campaigns and international campaigns. And with communication now being instant and available, all the groups plus any amount of individuals can all join forces when needs be.

It's a huge leap from the days of the suffragettes and even the feminists of the seventies who had to rely on the postal service, leaflets and posters, getting in the newspaper and preferably on TV (the seventies feminists not the suffragettes, who can only be admired for spreading the word so well in times of slow communication all round.) Now we can gather people together at the drop of a tweet and find out what's happening locally. Problem at work? Google it and there you are – someone twenty five miles away who's fought the same battle as you and can help you out. So no, I don't think there are too many campaigns and groups. But here's a few to whet your appetite.

POLITICAL PARTIES

You might want to sign up to a political party and see if you can't influence policies affecting older women from the powers in Westminster. Although at the time of writing, the liberal-conservative coalition is not all that active in this area. The conservatives are certainly setting policies on pensions and child care but then it's the women in between that we are concerning ourselves with here. The liberal website addresses some issues of concern, suggesting care credit for those who look after elderly relatives as well as caring for children. They propose well women clinics which will include support for women affected by family assault (domestic violence) and are also keen on caller ID to counteract the ten million obscene phone calls each year, which largely affect women. They are keen on flexible working too which certainly helps those in the sandwich generation.

However, the Clare Shaw award for getting older women well and truly on the political agenda goes to Labour. Harriet Harman started up the Labour Commission on Older Women and it's getting well and truly stuck into the issues. It was set up to look at three main issues – older women in the workplace, the caring responsibilities of older women and older women in public life. By older women they mean those between about 50 and 64, like Harriet Harman herself. Yes, Harriet is 63. I have to admit, I'd put her at about ten years younger than that and she certainly hasn't done an Anne Robinson.

I know I wrote a whole chapter about how it doesn't matter if you look your age and how we should not be made to feel we have to look younger and I stand by that. Still, well done Harriet. Why? Because most politicians of both sexes really age when they get into positions of power and responsibility and I like to think Harriet has learnt to pace herself and balance her life in a way that women tend to do so well. I also think she's an advocate for just making the most of yourself while not being all about how you look. I think I may be falling in love with Harriet Harman, or at least I think I've found a pretty good role model for how I want to be as an older woman. Should I get T shirts made up? Start a fan club? Try and get her to 'like' me on Facebook? I think not, but I will tell you about the first report from her commission on older women because it seems to be heading in the right direction.

In September 2013, the first report from this commission came out, identified some issues and made some useful initial suggestions. It found that unemployment among women between 50 and 64 had increased by 41% in the previous two and a half years. It recommended that all government funded schemes should support older women and that there should be a public debate about whether parental leave could be shared by grandparents. There's more in this report but this is not a manifesto for the labour party so look it up, keep an eye on this commission and nobble your MP if you want her or him to influence policy. As Yvette Cooper said – the generation of women who've broken glass ceilings and paved the way for their daughters and granddaughters deserve a better deal.

THE EVERYDAY SEXISM PROJECT

This was started by feminist writer, Laura Bates, in 2012 and has grown and grown into a very significant part of modern day feminism. You can upload your own examples of every day sexism as has happened to you onto their website or via Twitter. This is brilliant because it has posts from all over the world and from all ages. It has therefore helped this new wave of feminism become inclusive. It also takes small examples of sexism and when they are all added together, you get an accurate picture of our society today and what it means for women. So, when someone makes an inappropriate, sexist comment to you, then you have an answer to anyone who suggests you're making too much of it. Added with all the other comments, we can see a pattern and a culture that needs to keep changing. As an older woman, you might want to post some examples as they happen to you. There have been quite a few of these already, such as the older widow whose late husband's friends tried to pressurise her into sex. I have no idea how old the disabled woman was who was asked to pole dance around her walking stick, but it beggars belief. Show the world that misogyny affects all ages. So well done, Laura.

FEMINIST GROUPS

Google feminist groups and the name of your town and the chances are there are like minded women to meet up with. UK Feminista is an organisation which supports people to campaign for a world where men and women are equal. Just that. Simple but surely the bottom line – what we all want and need in this society. There are branches of Feminsta all over the country and the website supports anyone wanting to start a new group. I noted that in my home town, the local feminist group was based at our university. They mainly communicate on line and welcome those who are not at the Uni. Might just get an older woman's viewpoint in there.

FEMINIST BLOGS AND MAGAZINES

I suspect more of these will spring up over the next few months. At the moment, the main contenders are The Feminist Times, The F Word and The Vagenda. There are others tackling specific issues, such as Age At Work. It does keep you in touch with current issues and most are interactive so you can contribute with your comments too.

FUNDING

Fancy doing some research into attitudes towards older women? Fancy supporting older women in need? Rosa is a UK charitable fund for women and girls who might be able to support your project.

OTHER WOMEN'S GROUPS

There are groups for women who do not call themselves feminist groups but nevertheless provide a voice for women and are not immune to taking up the cause for feminists or for older women. The obvious example is the Women's Institute. This traditional 'Jam and Jerusalem' group has undergone a couple of revivals recently. First came the slow hand clapping of Tony Blair's speech in 2000, showing that the Institute was becoming more politicised. In 2012, the women's institute objected to an anti gay marriage advert, showing they are not afraid to get in there and fight for what's right. And yes, they will take on feminist matters too. The recent revival was when the organisation started to attract younger members and we now have meetings across the country where twenty, thirty, forty, fifty year olds and older women all meet together. And you know by now that I like the ages all mixed in and influencing each other.

Other women's organisations whether it's the Soroptomists or the Federation of Business and Professional Women or even your local book group bring together women of all ages. Feminism and older women issues are almost BOUND to be addressed at some point, even if that is not their primary remit. I like that. It reiterates the Every Day Sexism Project – things happen every day. Women are involved and concerned whether they are marching on Downing Street or sitting at a craft group. We should all be talking about it some of the time, we should all be aware of the issues all of the time.

There are bound to be issues that you feel particularly strongly about because THEY AFFECT YOU. It is likely that it will help you and others if you link up with women in the same boat. So if you are caring for an elderly relative, meet up with other carers, if you are forced into early retirement but want to carry on working, join a voluntary group or get together with others in your position to start up a business. Whatever your issue, there's bound to be a local group for you or an online forum to comment on.

THE UNIONS
In 2007, Sir Brendan Barber who was the General Secretary of the

TUC spoke at the Life Academy Annual Lecture, pointing out that ageism is the last respectable prejudice. He had a point and since then various trade unions have supported workers who have felt they've been discriminated against on the grounds of sex or age. Sir Brendan retired in 2012 when he was 61. Hopefully not pushed out of his job early by a young whippersnapper. While I'm flying the union flag, important guidelines were published by the TUC in 2011, outlining how union reps and employers should work together to support women through the menopause at work. This wasn't just some crazy union move to get men fanning women down in the lunch break, but was based on research published by the British Occupational Health Research Foundation in conjunction with the University of Nottingham. They found that basic understanding and practical support could make all the difference. They recommended simple things like plenty of ventilation and cool drinking water, toilets nearby and a greater understanding of menopausal related sick leave. Not rocket science really – I'm sure I could have come up with that without years of research. However, the important thing is the research led to a debate. And talking about this stuff is ALWAYS GOOD.

One piece of negativity concerning the unions came from Harriet Yeo, the outgoing chairman of Labour's executive committee. She said that unions were 'stuck in a time warp' and were dominated by male chauvinists obsessed with power games. If this is the case with your union, and it certainly isn't always so, the only way to change it is to become an active member.

There is one union I will give a special mention to – EQUITY. And not just because my actress daughter is a paid up member. In 2013, they called on the government to lead a crackdown on the use of female stereotypes in TV and theatre, suggesting that casting directors, agents, producers and directors should be encouraged to disregard female characters just based on attractiveness, caring responsibilities, or women as sex objects and victims. It certainly seems to me that you can't have a woman lawyer on TV, for example, without the script shouting out – ooh, look a female lawyer, how innovative! Or an older woman with a younger partner without some sort of titillation. So good on you, Equity. A way to go though. At the fifty year celebrations of the National Theatre only one female playwright was represented (mind you only 18% of their playwrights have been female since they started) and only 31.2% of the performers at the celebration were female. Oh very dear.

Interestingly, Belgium is ahead of us on this. Yes, Belgium – I knew they'd come up trumps eventually. They already have guidelines for broadcasters recommending they promote 'a balanced picture of diversity of roles and functions of men and women throughout programming' and to be 'vigilant with regard to sexual stereotyping.'

Problem at work? Get onto your union – they really can help. As can the citizen's advice bureau or firm of reputable lawyers, of course.

INTERNATIONAL GROUPS

Make yourself aware of what's happening around the world where women are often far more suppressed that in the West. Groups such as the Pink Gang in India use humour and wit to gain media coverage. They have, for example, painted their dogs pink and hung signs round them saying 'dog police' to make the point that they would make better policeman as at least they weren't corrupt and they could protect women against violence. And the women of Saudi Arabia, who defied a driving ban in a protest in October 13, deserve enormous respect as they were taking risks with the reduced liberty they already had as well as possibly facing harsh punishments.

MEN'S GROUPS AND CAMPAIGNS

Men want older women to be treated fairly and equally too. All right, not all men but THE VAST MAJORITY. Never before have so many men called themselves feminists and with many of them being older, they will support you in whatever battle you are fighting. Although this book is all about older women, men often become feminists from a young age and I am pleased to see that issues around sexism and respect for women are being addressed in our schools. There's an organisation run by men who go around schools carrying out workshops. Sounds great and I just love their name – GREAT MEN VALUE WOMEN. You can't say more than that.

It is really important that older women stand up and are counted. Some feminist issues don't affect me directly. Take FGM. I am not going to be faced with it and neither are my daughters. But it is happening to women out there and this is where the concept of sisterhood has to survive the 1970s and live on. My fellow women are being mutilated and I CARE. I might not be at the forefront of the campaign. But I have made myself knowledgeable about it and will spread that knowledge. I will sign any petition going and I will put my name to any protest.

Then there are the issues that affect me more directly. I am affected by not having older women role models on my TV screen, I am affected by being made to feel stupid by others just because of my age and sex and I am affected by magazines that airbrush every line out of an older woman's face so she looks like a plate. And I will shout about that too.

But one shout on its own can't be heard. A crowd shouting is better. And every woman on the planet shouting together is better still. So altogether now – AHHHGGGGGGG!

TEN: SEX WITHOUT PREJUDICE

I remember being a teenager when my mother hit forty. My father was one year older and as far as I was concerned, they were OLD and did not understand anything about anything, especially sex. Like each generation before mine, we all believed we invented sex and that our parents did some other old fashioned version of it, probably involving getting undressed in the dark, thinking of England and putting down a plastic protective sheet. As my mother told me about sex in such hushed tones I couldn't hear and involved her saying 'Don't get pregnant' over and over again, it's no surprise that I didn't equate the sexual act with the production of me. With some thought, I realised my parents must have done it three times (I have two older brothers) but I didn't want to dwell on that thought. Imagine my surprise then when as a teenager I discovered that my parents still had sex. It was a chance remark from my mother and I must have looked at her aghast because she said, 'of course we still, you know.' 'You know' was her phrase for sex, bless her.

I imagine nothing has changed and our children probably think we did it twice. They certainly won't want to think about it. Even worse, as a society we seem to put an age limit on sex. People just don't want to contemplate anyone over fifty having sex. Why is this? I suspect it has a lot to do with how sex is portrayed on film and TV. For one thing the couple are likely to be young and very, very attractive. The whole act will look perfect, as if choreographed by a ballet dancer. There won't be a fumble for contraceptives, they won't need to stop for the woman to point out that he hasn't quite found the right spot or to check that he'd put the rubbish out, and the phone won't ring in the middle of it all. Older couples are beginning to find their way as sexual beings onto our screens but it's still a novelty. No wonder a whole generation think that sex has an upper age of consent as well as a lower one.

It seems there has developed a sort of prejudice against older couples having sex. We never like to think of our parents having sex and have somehow transferred this to ALL older couples. Until we get older ourselves. Yuk, I used to say when I thought of women of my parents' age having sex. And no doubt the younger generation are now saying yuk about women of my age. It gets passed down from generation to generation and is exasperated by older women not feeling compelled to discuss it outside of their relationship. I wonder if this will change as the younger generation, who seem to discuss sex endlessly, get older. There are some changes though. Jane Fonda has written a book outlining positions for older couples to try. Shirley Conran writes a blog where sex is mentioned frequently which you might expect from the author of Lace. She makes it clear that even now she's in her eighties, she is still sexually active. I can't think of a British example off the top of my head. Funny that.

Let's get to the truth of the matter with the aid of some statistics. Saga, them with the holidays, carried out some useful research and discovered that 65% of over fifties are sexually active with 46% having sex at least once a week. 85% of those questioned said that sex was less pressurised than when they were younger, suggesting the quality was better. Bearing in mind the number of single older people, that's a pretty encouraging statistic.

I love a bit of research, especially where questionnaires are concerned. And when someone stops me in the street, I am quite disappointed when they only want to know if I shop from a catalogue. I'm still waiting for someone to surprise me and ask me when I last had sex. But some women have been asked this and other personal questions because research led by Linda J Waite of the University of Chicago in 2010 seems to support Saga's findings. This research found that in the 57-64 age group,

84% of men and 64% of women had had sex in the previous year. This fell to 38% of men and 17% of women in the 75-85 age group – not surprising as ill health becomes more prevalent after 80. In the 57-64 age group, 62% of men and 53% of women had oral sex. So good figures, but come on girls, let's get our quota up.

So, we're doing it but no one knows seems to be the message. I think the next generation down need to know that sexuality doesn't end in middle-age and get replaced with Mills and Boon books and Horlicks. However, I'm not suggesting you go to Speakers' Corner and shout out the details, or post on Facebook that you had a great session the night before. Like many of you, I consider sex to be the most personal of all things. Not because I'm coy or prudish but because this is intimate between me and my partner – just something for us and the thing that makes that relationship unique from other friendships. So no I won't be forcing the details on my younger friends, and guess what, I don't want to know the details of their personal intimacies either. Although occasionally I am given far too many details from an over confident twenty one year old I know.

I guess it's down to the arts and the media to get rid of the illusion that older women get their kicks from Bingo and a bar of Galaxy. So, all you authors out there, make sure the older woman character gets her pants off from time to time, all you playwrights, don't call your older woman character 'Mother', 'Grandmother' or 'Woman in the Supermarket.' Give her a name. And a sex life.

The reason for having a chapter on sex then is to help quell the stereotypes of the older woman and sexuality is part of that. We do have a voice, we do have a role to play in all aspects of society, we do want to be included and we are not a separate species. And part of this, is that we do have sex and we do fall in love. Young people don't have the monopoly on all of that.

The mathematicians among you will have noticed that

not 100% of over fifties are having sex. This is hardly surprising as many will have no partners and there are one or two barriers to sex as you get older which I will discuss later. (There are also some positives about sex over fifty which we will dwell on for some time). I remember the great, late Claire Rayner giving advice to an older woman – 'use it or lose it' (referring to sexuality). I was much younger at the time, but for some reason, it stuck in my head somewhere as I've just recalled that advice and it seems pretty sound. There are times in your life, when other things take over and sex takes a back seat. Having children is one of them when we can be too exhausted to even take our clothes off let alone indulge in some naked gymnastics. You just need to get back into the habit during that lull between toddler nightmares and teenagers out later than they promised. The same can happen as we get older. Something may have happened to get you out of the body bouncing routine – there is an increasing likelihood with age that you or your partner may go through a period of ill health, or undergo a bereavement, or suffer from anxiety of even depression. But Claire was right – use it or lose it. Get back in the saddle (not literally unless of course you get turned on by the smell of Dubbin on leather). We just have to put our minds to it, and our bodies, I suppose.

In case you are looking for good reasons to re-start the middle-aged bedroom Olympics, take a look at my list.

1.   Women with an active sex life live longer.
2.   Research suggests regular sex can make you look younger. I know I said it wasn't important but still...
3.   Sex can make you fitter and uses a fair amount of calories.
4.   Sex helps keep your relationship fresh.
5.   Having a good physical relationship helps boost your confidence.
6.   It's better than Eastenders (usually).

We know there are health, well being and psychological benefits to an active sex life but as you get older there are barriers. However, the good news is that all those barriers can be overcome. So, a list of barriers, focusing on the ones most likely to affect older women.

1. YOU'VE GOT OUT OF THE HABIT

We've discussed this already but it happens. If that's all that's wrong, get back into the habit. This may mean making yourself have sex when you're not sure if you feel like it. This is completely different to your partner making you have sex which is never acceptable. But it's as easy to get out of the sex habit as it is to get out of the habit of putting the bins out on a Thursday when they change it from Wednesday. Maybe I shouldn't liken sex to putting out the bins although there's a certain satisfaction from both activities.

2. MENOPAUSAL SYMPTOMS

The menopause is such a big issue for many middle-aged women that it has a chapter later. But there is no doubt that hormonal changes can lead to a loss of libido. However, it's important not to blame it on the hormones if it could be something else entirely. Maybe you've had a change in your lifestyle, maybe you've got out of the habit as described earlier, maybe you haven't been well. Rule everything out first and then discuss it with your GP. Some women swear by HRT, while others prefer to give it a miss. Discuss the pros and cons and then make the right decision for you. But remember that you can go on having a great sex life after the menopause. It's possible you might go off it temporarily but never see the menopause as the end of the line. A lot of women surveyed have gone on to describe how sex is, in fact, better after the menopause. Make sure it isn't just that YOU EXPECT IT TO ALL GO DOWNHILL IN THE MENOPAUSAL

YEARS. Someone (probably your mother) may have told you it's all over with your first grey hair or hot flush but it isn't. Don't be swayed by what is little more than an old wives' tale. No one is saying you have to be swinging from the chandeliers in a wonder woman costume, but don't rush into giving it up completely.

3. LESS MOBILITY
It may be that you or your partner have less mobility than you used to. Work round it. Some older women have said that sex gets better because they have to be more creative and inventive to make it work for them. There are self help books out there on this so get to your library.

4. POOR HEALTH
As you get older, there is an increased chance that you may have periods of poor health but you may not. My own parents were fit and healthy and reasonably mobile into their eighties. I don't want to think about whether they had an active sex life – we still don't like to imagine our parents, however old we are. So yes, you may stop or slow up during periods of poor health but if it's something you will get better from, then keep it on your to do list for later. Keep the home fires burning, as they say.

5. ERECTILE DYSFUNCTION
This is one of the main causes of sexual problems in older men. It does not affect all men by any means – it really is the minority. Nevertheless, if it happens to your partner, you are not alone. And if you go to your GP to discuss it, she or he will have seen it all before and heard many similar stories. And guess what, doctors aren't any more embarrassed about it than if you had an in-growing toenail. So don't you be. IT CAN BE SORTED. With medication, in some instances. In other cases it may be due to other heath issues or even depression BUT YOU CAN BE

HELPED. The main reason for not seeking help is embarrassment, or men who quite simply don't like going to the doctors. Suggest you go with him, although some men prefer to go by themselves and that's fine too. Suggest he writes the problem down and hands it to the doctor. So much better than turning up, losing his bottle and pretending he came to have his ear syringed. And yes, look at the internet if only to see it's a common complaint and to get you into discussing it between you before approaching a third party.

6. VAGINAL DRYNESS AND SORENESS

One word – LUBRICATE. Go to your pharmacist. Don't want to shout the details out in front of a queue which will inevitably contain a selection of neighbours, colleagues and someone you like to flirt with? Then choose a chemist where you can ask to see the pharmacist privately - and most of them have this facility. Or just pick something up off the shelves. Once again, remember you are not alone. Studies suggest 20% of menopausal women have problems with lubrication and 14% have some pain with sex which might be the same thing so off to your pharmacist or doctor, it's just another routine job. You wouldn't expect an engine to run without oil. You wouldn't expect to make decent pastry without margarine. And you wouldn't expect to get down the flume without water.

7. YOU CAN'T TALK ABOUT IT ANY MORE

Or maybe you never really have talked about it. For some couples, it's all just flowed naturally and your non-verbal responses and cries of ecstasy have said it all. No need to have the 'how was it for you' conversation afterwards. Then you get older and you suddenly need to say 'mind me bad leg' or 'I'll need a bit of lubrication' but you're not used to these more direct conversations. Well, have a conversation about having a conversation if you like. Or just say it. It may be that you've changed partners later in life and whereas it all went without saying the first time round, your new partner needs a bit of, well, guidance. IS IT REALLY WORTH BEING QUIET ABOUT IT AND MAKING HIM THINK ALL IS PERFECT UNDER THE DUVET? No, of course not. And the longer you leave it, the harder it will be (if you get my drift). If you wait six months before saying, 'that doesn't really do it for me,' then not only have you wasted six months of what could have been earth moving, but your new partner will be rather confused and possibly upset.

If you find it hard to talk about all matters intimate because it's a new need for you, then you will have to make yourself. You may prefer to talk to a girlfriend first. Or even say it out loud to yourself (though not when walking round the library or anything.) Just hearing yourself saying the words you want to say will make it easier because you will realise that it's easy. It's just saying one word after the other really. And think of the results. It could make the difference between a revived sex life and a dwindling one.

8. MENTAL HEALTH ISSUES

Older women are prone to mental health problems, including depression. There's been a surge in other mental health issues in middle-aged women, such as eating disorders. The cause is unclear but there is no doubt the pressures of living are greater than ever. There is no time here to go into the problems you may encounter but undoubtedly mental health issues, particularly depression, do have an adverse effect on sex. Obviously. If you don't even feel like getting out of the bed in the morning, you're hardly going to feel like bouncing on the bed at night. You'll need to get treatment and put sex on hold until you are up to it. And be mindful that men are less open about mental health issues. You may be the first to notice that your partner is depressed. And one of the signs may be that he loses libido. Get him to get help, while remembering that any sexual problems affect both of you - deal with them as a couple. And remember, when your fully blown, fully penetrative sex life has to be on hold, don't stop being intimate altogether. STILL HAVE A CUDDLE. In fact lots of them. It's very comforting and very therapeutic.

9. YOU'RE TOO TIRED
This is apparently the top reason given by older women for not getting the duvet creased. Might be worth getting a blood test to check your iron. Heavier periods as menopause approaches often result in some anaemia which will inevitably lead to feeling tired. So find out if you need to be taking an iron supplement. And then look at your routines. Kids left home? Then why wait until the late evening? Retired or working more flexible hours now? Then start the day with a bang.

10. GUILT
This can happen to women who have had a long term partner who dies. Moving on to a new partner can lead to guilt when trying to have an intimate relationship, and this can really stop a woman from enjoying sex. Bereavement counselling can help or just talking to a close friend or family member. They will all tell you that you deserve a sex life, that your first partner would want you to have fun and that sex is very healing.

BUT THE GOOD NEWS IS...
Sex can often get better in later years. Once you realise that Hollywood has got it all wrong – sex is not just for the young and beautiful - then you can lie back (or any way you want) and enjoy it.
1. Let's remind ourselves that Saga found 85% of older people said sex is less pressurised than when they were younger.

2. According to the Sexual Advice Association, women often have quicker arousal post menopause. They suggest this may be connected with a reduced risk of pregnancy. (By the way it is recommended that you use contraception for a year after your periods stop or two years if you are under fifty).

3. Older women feel freer now the children have left home. Any room, any time, any how. The only interruption is likely to be a son or daughter phoning for a loan.

4. Older women know what they like. If you tried it in the wardrobe in 1988 and didn't like it then, chances are you still won't want to involve furniture. If you are in a long term relationship, you will know each other's bodies and be very familiar with what turns each other on. So much better than those poor young things still trying to feel their way. Celebrate your mutual knowledge.

5. Having a new partner will make you feel young and loved all over again.

This is all very lovely. You now know that you can get older disgracefully, you can enjoy sex until you drop and the chances are it will be even better than before. Great. What's not to like? However, we cannot isolate ourselves from what is happening in the rest of society. I have already advocated exchanging views and advice with the young, mixing up the ages and paying minimal attention to the date of birth on your passport. We live in a society where there are some questionable things going on when it comes to sex. Our children are becoming sexualised at a younger age, young boys are learning about sex via bad porn on the internet – the sort where women are demeaned and controlled. Cyber bullying often involves persuading vulnerable young girls to photo or film themselves indulging in sexual acts and the internet is awash with sexual predators including paedophiles.

My first reaction to all this is to say 'Phew, thank God I'm in my fifties and my children are confident young women in their twenties and I've just been reading I can carry on having the sex life I want indefinitely.' But WE ARE ALL PART OF THIS SOCIETY and so the problem is everyone's.

If you have young daughters you will obviously want to talk to them about on line safety and sex in general. You will need to make sure they can talk openly to you about anything that might go wrong in their life. And if you can talk about sex openly, honestly and using all the words (not euphemisms or coyly avoiding anything too near the mark) then she will find it easier to talk to you. And if you are a teacher or youth worker, you will need to do the same with the kids you work with – you may be the one person that teenager or young woman feels she can talk to. For years my mother talked about 'down below' and it confused me greatly – I thought she was talking about something she'd buried in the garden. Say vagina, penis, penetration and whatever else you want to say. You really don't want to be saying 'pushing the train into the sidings' or other such confusing nonsense.

Having said all that, it is going to be the young person's peer group who will be the best support. You can make yourself available, you can mop up the tears, but it isn't going to be older people who change sexual bullying, inappropriate porn and objectification of young girls. It has been shown that the best way of tackling bullying in general has been to set up peer support and I believe this is needed to tackle the growing menace of sexual bullying. So if you are working with young people, try and get this set up. Young people who have been victims might be prepared to speak out to others, young people who are having problems might find it easier to talk to their peers, and on line forums to discuss all this stuff cannot be run by a fifty year old woman who looks like she might be out of touch, even if she isn't.

The truth is we will be out of touch. As soon as one website is identified as being a source of bullying, another one is set up. They pop up on a daily basis. When you are a teenager you are sex curious so boys will look at porn – maybe we should make sure they see good porn where women are not seen as victims of humiliation, even rape. Many young people have two accounts on social networking sites – one their parents can see and another private one. Teenagers are trying to break away and part of that is breaking the rules and not sharing things with their parents. So there will be a limit to what adults can do. So help by proxy – through other young people in the know.

MICHAEL GOVE SYNDROME

If you are going to play any part at all in changing the culture for younger people, then you need to be in touch with what young people want, how they behave and what's going on in the world for them. When he was education secretary, Michael Gove suggested that young people texted poetry to each other instead of pictures of their or girls' private parts. Yea, right, as if that's all it takes – someone like Michael Gove to make a suggestion. He might also try asking them to ditch the vodka mixes and go for a Ribena. Or give up going out on a Saturday and have a nice early night. There are some cool older people who could helpfully make suggestions – more likely to be a rap artist than a politician. Particularly a politician like Michael Gove who is, in my opinion, about as much in touch with young people as a Buddhist monk on a thirty year retreat. So if you're cool – get in there and if you are not, then helping the young to help the young could be the best thing you could do. Young people may have reason to think we are not much better than Michael Gove – after all, we didn't go through cyber bullying or boys texting us pictures of their penises and all the rest of this internet sexual stuff. By the way, other things you need to know about Michael Gove were reported by the New Statesman and include the fact that he has as many pictures of Margaret Thatcher in his office as his wife and children. He also finds Angela Merkel 'hot'. I feel I should like him for flying the flag of older women.(But I just can't).

GOING SOLO

We've talked about mid life sex as if all women have a partner on hand and all they need to do is get him/her out of the potting shed and into bed. However, there are more single older women than ever before. Some have always been single and this number is increasing and some find themselves single having previously been in a relationship.

SWOFTIES

Or single women over fifty. This includes still singles, widows and divorcees, and swofties are rising in number. There are now well over 600,000 of them and it seems that they are having a good time. 1,000 of them were interviewed for a survey commissioned by the Department of Work and Pensions and a quarter of them reported that they were the happiest they've ever been. Half were learning a new skill, a quarter had joined a gym and 20% reported a very active social life. 17% percent of those surveyed were actively dating. Sounds good although there's not much substance here. What about the three quarters, for example, who did NOT report it was the happiest time of their life. Presumably plenty of them were still happy but had not quite topped that Eric Clapton concert in the 1970s. While others, for all we know, might be downright miserable. Some will have chosen to be on their own while others will have found themselves on their own by chance or misfortune. So I decided to conduct my own mini survey. This was hardly scientific and just involved me chatting to the thirty single over fifties I knew. The result is stating the bleeding obvious – those who have made the choice to be single are very happy and those who were forced into it via bereavement or unwanted divorce/separation were not as happy. No wonder the surveys are largely inconclusive if they lump all single older women in together. There is not a one size fits all view of this.

FREEMALES
The number of women who have never married or had children has doubled over the last three decades. Some date, some don't but either way, the majority report high levels of happiness. Many have always lived alone and so have not had to adjust to a partner leaving and/or the kids flying the nest.

I still remember a time when marriage followed by children, with a career taking second place was the expectation for most women. Now, women have the full range of lifestyle choice without an expectation of being judged for their choice. I am not claiming that there is no judgement, but there is not the expectation of it. Same sex relationships, long term relationships with or without marriage, second, third or fourth marriages, living with friends, single parents, living with adult children or living alone. All good ways to live your life. It has to be a better society where there are more choices for women and there should, theoretically, be a greater chance of finding happiness because of it. However, there are plenty of single older women out there who would prefer to have a long term partner and the majority of them claim that meeting that significant partner gets harder as you get older.

DATING AS YOU GET OLDER
When you suddenly find yourself single in later life, you may be so scared at the prospect of dating again that you rush out and buy three dogs, a cat and a budgie and hope that will satisfy your

need for companionship. Trouble is, it won't satisfy any physical desire (at least I hope it doesn't). The chances are you will get plenty of encouragement from friends and family so if you think you want a new partner, then take a deep breath and get dating. There's no other way for it. You need to meet someone, get to know them and hope you click and that process is dating. You can't get a man out of a catalogue – even if you find someone on line, you'll still need to do the dating bit.

Most of the research into how we meet partners has been carried out in America. Maybe they're nosier than we are, though I doubt it. Anyway, I suspect dating habits in the USA are pretty similar to here. Just with less meeting in pubs and more analysis. A survey by Dr Gian Gonzaga for eHarmony did not find much difference across the ages. All ages found the biggest percentage of people met at educational establishments or work, followed by through friends and family. Then on line dating, then bars clubs and social events followed by 'other' and finally through a church or religious place. For older couples the order was exactly the same, just slight adjustments in the percentages. I found myself wondering about the 8.8 of people who met through 'other' means.   At first it sounded all rather weird but then I remembered some of my friends who met in unusual ways. My favourite was a colleague who met her partner when she fell off a bus, closely followed by a couple I know who met when she went round to his flat to borrow a cup of sugar. Mind you, she'd tried nearly every flat in a huge complex until she got a hit.

Other Unusual Places Women Have Met A Partner
1.   In the Gents. (She was desperate and it was empty, at least when she went in.)
2.   Hiding from the ticket man in a train toilet (there's a theme here)
3.   Climbing a tree (honestly!)

4. Pretending to have a stammer to meet a particular speech therapist.
5. On a roller coaster.
6. At the council rubbish tip.
7. In Greggs
8. After getting a foot stuck in a man hole.
9. After falling asleep on a bed in a furniture showroom.
10. Getting lost after getting off in the middle of a ghost train ride.

Going back to the research, I was pleased that dating isn't that different whatever your age. Obviously, the older you are, the more experienced you are so you don't have that fear of the first time. Nevertheless, we meet people in very similar ways and there's no doubt the feelings are very much the same. Older people do complain that it's harder to meet someone as you age and there is a certain amount of truth in that. For one thing, we are less likely to be in education which is a very popular meeting ground. And we may have been in the same job for longer and already discovered that Richard from accounts is to be avoided and if Dean's hovering by the water dispenser, opt for intense dehydration. It could be argued that older women are less likely to go into bars but that's a matter of personal taste. It seems older men still like to go into pubs, clubs and bars so if it's something you want to do and if you're looking to meet someone, don't rule it out.

However, meeting a partner is often something that happens when you're busy doing other things. If you happen to be in a bar having a good time with friends then you're going to have a good evening whether or not you meet someone else. If you set out purely to meet someone and you don't, then you'll probably consider the evening to be a waste of time and a failure. So do join clubs, do indulge in your hobbies and interests and do, well, get out there. If you've been in the same circle of friends for years, then you will have to meet new people. So have the aim of meeting new people and take it from there. You might end up with some good new friends of both sexes and if Mr or Ms Wright comes along, then great. The main thing to remember is that you are not going to meet someone sitting at home watching Homes Under The Hammer. You might meet someone at home on your laptop, mind you.

INTERNET DATING

One in five relationships now starts on line and this is set to increase. Some predict it will move on up to number two or even number one on the list of places we meet our partner. And the number of over forties involved in internet dating has risen sharply. There are now a number of dating websites specialising in older people – whether it's over forties, over fifties or beyond. Older women have traditionally been a bit averse to online dating but this is rapidly changing.

If you are single and the thought of internet dating makes you cringe and shout 'It's not normal' or 'It's for sad, lonely people,' then question your reaction. Back when you first dated, there was no internet dating. I suppose the equivalent was putting a 'would like to meet' advert in the local paper. And it was a minority who advertised. So yes, it wasn't the norm. But it is now. So not everyone on line is sad and lonely and anyway WHAT IF THEY ARE. If you've lost a partner or a partner has moved on, it would be perfectly normal to feel a bit sad and lonely from time to time. If you've questioned your aversion to internet dating and you still feel that you'd rather be stuck in a lift for twenty four hours with Michael Gove and Godfrey Bloom, then fine. Do whatever's right for you. There are no dos and don'ts. Actually there are, especially when 'meeting' someone on line.

INTERNET DO'S AND DON'TS

Once again, these are pretty similar to the dos and don'ts whatever your age. You may think the older you are, the wiser you are to dating traps. Not necessarily. We may worry about young girls being 'groomed' by older men claiming to be teenagers, but you too can be taken in by an out of date photo of a single man who's helpfully hiding his wedding ring finger under the desk. Whatever your age, YOU DON'T KNOW FOR CERTAIN who you are talking to. So here's the list:

1. Be honest in your own profile. You don't want to be retracting your high flying job later when you turn up to meet him with your Greggs name badge on.

2. Make your profile interesting and avoid clichés. Do you really long for cosy nights in by a log fire? And does that make you sound any different from all those other women who like log fires. An alien logging into one of these websites will conclude that we are a nation tied to the hearth rug. And anyway, men might interpret cosy nights in rather differently from you. And don't state the obvious – no one ever thinks they have no sense of humour, even if they clearly haven't. So SHOW you have a sense of humour with a witty line, and if your interests really are going for walks in the country and reading, then put some stuff you'd like to try as well.

3. Learn to interpret his profile. If you think 'looking for fun' means a day out at a theme park, you are probably too naïve to be on a dating site. Possibly to be dating.

4. Spend some time 'talking' on line before meeting. You will get a sense of whether the person is likely to be suitable. If he just agrees with everything you say and likes exactly the same things as you, be wary.

5. Once you know his full name, Google it. If he tells you where he works, check it out – but quietly and anonymously if

possible. Best not to turn up there asking for ID.

6. Back more than one horse. The one who seems ideal could turn out to be married, twenty years older than his photos suggests. Or Michael Gove. Chat to any of interest and take time before you dismiss any of them. Unless he states early on that he likes quiet nights in with his train set while the woman of his dreams whips him up a mushroom omelette.

7. Be cynical to the point of being wise. But remember too that many relationships start on line and carry on happily. Sometimes ever after. So be cynical but not too cynical. Wise, though, always wise.

8. So, you've 'chatted' on line and you think this could work. Ideally have a phone conversation next. You might want to disguise your number by dialling 141 first. Just in case. You might even want a separate pay as you go phone. Just in case. Or you might want to skip the phoning and go straight to a meet up. But you can tell a fair amount about someone on the phone – more than on line as tone of voice indicates a whole range of things – age, attitude, class (if that's important) and sex (if that's important.)

9. Which reminds me – you might have started out with a description of the partner who you think would be ideal for you. This could include physical appearance, type of job, whether or not he has children, interests and so on. Go through it again and whittle it down to what's ESSENTIAL. Does it really matter if he's half an inch shorter? Does it matter what kind of job he does? Maybe it does and that's fine. But I ended up with someone who didn't tick many of my original boxes. He was tall, slim and good looking so he ticked that box (sorry John – IS tall, slim and good looking.) But he did a job I thought boring, was older than me and a couple of other items I had thought incompatible. Yet, we clicked straight away and have been clicking ever since. So

don't restrict yourself too much by ideals. Sometimes we don't know our ideal until we are face to face with it.

10. So you think you want to meet. He's clearly lovely and completely trustworthy so why not invite him round for a cosy dinner? NO! Apply a principle here called 'WHAT WOULD I SAY TO MY DAUGHTER?' The cautions you would discuss with her about meeting someone she had come across on line apply to you. Obviously. And yet older women are often not as cautious as they should be. Meet on neutral territory, don't go for an expensive meal or night out at the theatre on a first date but start with a drink or a coffee. Arrange your transport home in advance and don't give away personal details like your address until you are sure of him. You may want to have friends sitting on the other side of the café or bar. You can ask a friend to phone you an hour in so you can say 'I've got to go, something urgent's come up.' OK, you will both know it's pre-arranged but it saves any embarrassment or you trying to squeeze out of the toilet window.

I feel like going off on a tangent here. Just to remind you that you're a feminist. You believe in equal opportunities for women and a society that treats everyone with respect. And ideally, you want to meet a man who is also a feminist. More men openly call themselves feminists while others are feminists who just don't realise it. The men who believe in equality and treating all women with respect, men who never objectify women and who abhor those who do. But they don't realise the word 'feminist' applies to them. Don't worry about the semantics – you can explain all of that later. In the meantime, avoid the following:

1. Men who say ask you to iron their shirts on the second date.
2. Men who use patronising expressions such as 'don't worry

your pretty little head about that.'

3. Men who ask the size of your breasts but never ask what you do as a job.

I could go on but I think this is best illustrated with some concrete examples.

So, personally, I wouldn't get a date with someone like:

1. Godfrey Bloom (Former UKIP MEP)

Why?

Because 1. He made a comment about women not cleaning behind the fridge as being sluts. 2. He referred to third world countries as 'bongo bongo land.' 3. He said 'No self-respecting small business man with a brain in the right place would ever employ a lady of child bearing age.' 4. When given a place on the European Parliaments' women's rights committee (!), said 'I am here to represent Yorkshire women who always have the dinner on the table when you get home.' 5. His website states that his hobbies are hunting and shooting .

2. David Gilmour (Canadian Author and university professor)

Why?

Because 1. He states he won't teach books written by women or Chinese authors. 2. He states he hasn't come across any female authors he is passionate about to teach (although he does teach one of Virginia Woolf's short stories). 3. Maybe he hasn't heard of Jane Austen, the Bronte's, Margaret Atwood etc. By the way, he is not to be confused with Pink Floyd's David Gilmour who I would definitely date if only to listen to him playing the guitar as only he can.

3. Rush Limbaugh (America radio talk show host)

Why?

Because 1. He said of Hilary Clinton 'all she is is a secretary.' 2. He called a law student a slut for advocating cheaper contraceptives. 3. When racing car driver, Danica Patrick spoke out on the same topic, he said 'what do you expect from a woman driver.' 4. Of author, Tracie McMillan who wrote a book about healthy eating, he said 'What is it with all you single, white women.' 5. He said that feminism was established so as to allow unattractive women easier access to the mainstream of society. Nice.

4. Silvio Berlusconi (Italian Politician)

Why?

No explanation needed but try these quotes for size – 1. Another reason to invest in Italy is that we have beautiful secretaries – superb girls. 2. When asked if they would like to have sex with me, 30% said 'yes' while the other 70% said 'what again?' 3. It's better to have a passion for beautiful girls than to be gay.

5. Jerry Lewis (Comedian)

Why? Here he is in action – 'I don't like any female comedians. A woman doing comedy doesn't offend me, but sets me back a bit. I, as a viewer, have trouble with it. I think of her as a producing machine that brings babies in the world.'

6. AA Gill.

Why?

Do you have to ask...?

None of these are online but just a warning that there are others in that vein. Avoid, that's all I'm saying.

So, you've been on a date and it went well. More than well, you really want to see him again. And you do. So, what's the problem? We know that the course of true love never did run smooth, as Shakespeare would have us know. And the problems and potential hiccups are mostly the same whatever age you are. But let's look at some of the barriers to true love which are more pertinent in middle-age and beyond:

1. MEET THE CHILDREN

It's no longer meet the parents which might cause some anxiety, but meet the children. His/hers and yours. The first decision you will need to make is when is it timely to do the 'this is my new…?' speech. Notice how I haven't put boyfriend because even the terminology is wrought with problems. When, if ever, are you too old to say 'boyfriend?' (or girlfriend). Does man friend sound a bit Robinson Crusoe? Does 'friend' really convey what you want to convey or will your children just think you've met someone to go to bingo with? Does 'partner' suggest he or she has got his/her suitcases and furniture in the car and will soon be monopolising the remote control? There are no easy answers, although I would avoid 'lover', at least to start with. Many women prefer to just use his name as in 'I'd like you to meet Simon' and when pressed say that he is a special friend. Sounds a bit Enid Blyton school story but it's not bad. You may find your child will start to say a word herself such as boyfriend and you can take her (or his) lead.

Having sorted out the terminology, you will need to decide when and how. This will depend on the age of your children, whether they are still getting over the break with their father, their personalities, whether they are in the middle of important exams – all manner of things. So there is not going to be an easy guide here. No rules such as 'tell your children after the third date' or 'tell your children when you are absolutely positive this is for life.'

However, here are a few things to think about:
1. With older children you can approach the subject before you even think about dating. Ask them if they think it's a good idea (if you're fairly sure they'll say yes) and they might even help you. Then when you meet 'the one' it won't exactly come as a surprise.
2. Younger children may prefer the 'special friend' description, along with bucketfuls of reassurance that they remain as

important to you as ever.

3. Remember though that you are entitled to a love life so, while being sensitive to your children's emotional needs, there is no need to put it off until they have left home and have children of their own.

4. Pick your time for telling them. Not to be blurted out in the middle of an argument so it looks like it's a punishment for them. And not during other stressful times in their life (in the middle of exams, when they've just split up with a boy/girlfriend etc)

5. If they are sensitive and likely to find the whole scenario very difficult then you may want to put off telling them until you are sure it's serious or likely to be. What's the point (unless they are more directly involved as in point one) in telling them you are hoping to start a new life with Clive when you've only chatted on the phone to find your date ruined by his sexist remarks, halitosis and insistence on showing you his in-growing toenail.

6. If they have a strong relationship with their father, reassure them that no one is going to replace their Dad.

It's common sense really and standing back and trying to see things from your child's point of view. If your children are adults, they can be just as sensitive but it's even more important to remember that you deserve a relationship, if that's what you want. There's nothing as bad as a thirty year old having a tantrum because her mother has the audacity to be unavailable for babysitting because she's dating.

As for meeting his children, just remember that they may be wary of you so DON'T TRY TOO HARD. You don't have to love them, but you do have to accept that they will be part of his life and if don't want his baggage then find someone with better baggage.

2. FINANCIAL CONCERNS

I am not one to give financial advice as my way of budgeting is to spend my money until the bank tells me I haven't got any more (no wonder my daughters struggle.) But clearly you won't want to rush into a joint bank account on the second date. And make sure your will is up to date. If you want your savings to go to your children, even if you re-marry, then make sure you've done the legalities. And I don't have to remind you of the many stories where women have trusted the untrustworthy and lost their life savings.

3. UNKNOWN PASTS

When you meet someone in your twenties, you can pretty well go through your past loves in the time it takes to drink three vodka tonics. Later you can fill in the important bits of your childhood and you're done. The older you are, the more there is to reveal and it will take you longer to find out everything you need to know about a potential partner. So what do you actually need to know? You may want to ask about how many times the guy has been married. You may think it's a bad sign if he's been married more than five times for example. Or you may not care one way or the other. Or you may want to know whether he has a criminal record. What's important will be different for everyone but it's worth deciding what you want to ask directly. It's easy to hear a lot of memories about his holidays and school days and think you know all you need to know. Dig deep if you need to.

4. DO I KNOW WHAT TO DO?

This sounds like the cry of a teenager but if you've been with the same partner for years and are starting again, it will feel like you've gone back to the beginning. You may have got used to saying 'Have you got put the dishwasher on?' in the middle of sex which is not quite so acceptable the first time with someone new.

Or you may even find yourself both wanting to sleep on the left hand side of the bed. There will be a lot a readjusting and that's fine. Just be honest and tell him about your fears and uncertainties. You're not a teenager so no need to try and blag it.

5. WHAT IF I'M MAKING A HUGE MISTAKE

Take it one step at a time, proceed with caution and if it turns out to be a mistake then laugh, learn and move on.

6. SHOULD I GIVE UP AND TAKE UP KNITTING?

Only if you want to. It's ok to feel scared, uncertain, doubtful and every other emotion there is. If you want to give it a go, give it a go and if you really don't, then don't. No expectations from others, from you or from society. We really do have the whole range of choice available to us now.

DO I HAVE TO?

No. There are no rules which say you have to get a partner, no rules which dictate you should want a partner. Many people go solo and love it. A third of us live on our own now. If that's you, then great. You can have a perfectly happy, active and fulfilling life living by yourself. Check your own honesty to make sure you are not opting out because you're a bit scared or because you think it's the easy option. If you still come to the conclusion that life for you is better on your own then great. It's all about finding what works for you. And remember, there is no shame in changing your mind. A few thoughts:-

1. Don't be pressurised by other people.

Friends may be very well meaning when they set you up on a date with Gerry from accounts. They may not take any notice of your mild protestations. So be firm. Explain that you want to be alone and that you really want to be included in any event, dinner party, trip to the zoo, whatever BUT WITHOUT A POTENTIAL

PARTNER YOU DON'T WANT. If they still don't listen, write a letter on proper paper, put it in a proper envelope, stick a proper stamp on it and post it in a proper post box. Of course you can chat, email, tweet or stand on a hill and say it in semaphore. But a proper letter is often good for something that comes from the heart. It tends to be taken seriously. If necessary point out that it hurts you to think people only take you seriously if you are one of a pair.

2. Set the trend for group events where not everyone is a couple.

There is still a trend to invite pairs of people to dinners or events as if you are somehow not complete on your own. So set the trend for how you want things to be by hosting a dinner party for couples and you, or maybe couples and some singles but where it's clear you are not pairing anyone up. Brothers maybe or gay and straight mixes. That way your friends who are a couple hopefully won't think twice about inviting you as a complete package on your own.

3. Friends will be even more important.

Unless you want to live a life as a recluse (and yes, that's a valid option too) you will find that good friends are essential. There's an old saying which suggests that to have a good friend, you have to be a good friend and that's so true. Keep in touch with old friends in whatever way you can and make new friends by chatting to anyone and everyone. Be assertive. If you find yourself chatting to someone at the swimming pool, then suggest a coffee afterwards. You have to work hard at friendships and put the time and effort in. Just like romantic relationships, you get out of it what you put in. Oh and family's included here so be a good aunt, cousin, daughter etc.

4. Go out alone.

There are no rules which state that you can't go to the cinema, theatre, restaurant or anywhere on your own. You may find it seems more acceptable to go to some activities than others. Most women wouldn't think twice about going solo to a class at the gym, or signing up for an educational course of some sort. So why not go to a film you really want to see on your own? It's not as if you need someone to chat to during the screening (although I often seem to sit in front of those that do.) And you don't need to shout out as you arrive 'I am not sad, I do have friends but I really wanted to see this film and no one was available.' Of course you're not sad, you are simply confident enough to go on your own if that's what you fancy doing.

5. It's not written in stone.

Living alone may be perfect now and it may be perfect for the next ten years and beyond. But it's fine to change your mind. Even if you have spent the last twenty years telling everyone how happy you are on your own. You can be happy on your own AND STILL find happiness hitched up with someone else.

6. Alone or something else.

There are other choices of course. You can share with friends, relatives, live in a commune, travel round the country/world with no fixed abode, live with seventy pets. I cannot say it enough times – *THERE ARE NO RULES.*

So there we have it. We've talked about having sex, not having sex, living the lifestyle that's right for you and not dating Michael Gove. (Apart from anything, his wife may have something to say about that.) As with everything, there's a big overlap with things that affect the younger generation and there are some things which are specific to the older generation. One of these is dealing with an emptying nest (or changes in the nest). Hankies at the ready for the next chapter.

ELEVEN: THE CHANGING LOOK OF YOUR NEST

When you have children, you know somewhere at the back of your mind that one day they will grow up and leave home. But it's tucked away right back far from any conscious thought. There with the knowledge that we're all going to die, that there will always be an argument with someone at Christmas and that if you come out of the toilets with your skirt tucked in your knickers, there will be at least one person you want to impress watching you. Things we never ever think about until they happen. So, when your offspring tells you the date she's leaving for Uni, a new flat or travelling you will be completely taken by surprise. Believe me, it will creep up on you like yet another new series of X factor. And you won't be prepared. Even though you might have had to wait some time for the big exit. And even though the big exit may be followed a year or so later by the big entrance. Yes, I'm talking adults who never seem to leave like Ronnie Corbett in 'Sorry', and the boomerang kids who bounce back when their overdraft reaches its limits.

WHEN?

In these austerity days when rent and the price of everything is rocketing, the average age for leaving home is twenty seven. And there are an awful lot of thirty and forty year olds still in the bedroom with 'WENDY'S ROOM' and 'KEEP OUT' on the door. And when children leave home for university, chances are they'll come back older and poorer and with three years worth of washing.

If we define adult children as the over twenties, then more than three million of them live with parents, according to the office of national statistics. There are more males (1.8 million) than females (1.1 million) and it is suggested that mothers tend to molly coddle boys more, picking up their dirty pants and collecting their crusted mugs every day. So maybe the boys value the laundry and meals service more than their freedom. The number of overgrown kids living in the shadow of their mother's washing machine is rising. There were 20% more of them in 2013 than in 1997. The next generation will probably watch an old episode of Friends and wonder where the parents are. Perhaps the washing machine has broken and they're at the launderette.

WHY?

The main reason, as you would expect, is financial. Rents have soured, students have huge debts when they graduate, there is high unemployment among young people – no wonder they are coming home to roost. Many young people have no choice – they either move back home (or don't leave in the first place) or get further into debt. Others see it as a way forward, paying little or no rent to enable them to save for a deposit on a flat.

In many ways, this seems like a sensible and logical decision. There are disadvantages, of course. We want our children to learn to live independently and living at home doesn't really do the job, but still it's unlikely to be permanent. As a short term fix, you can't fault it. Other reasons are a reluctance to break away or just a realisation that life at home is more comfortable and convenient, particularly if Mum or Dad is doing all the cooking and cleaning. In this case, you might want to have what I call a 'long chat.' IF YOUR CHILD CAN AFFORD TO LEAVE HOME THEN THIS IS WHAT SHE SHOULD DO. If it's fear, then see if you can talk it through, make it gradual so they come home for weekends, reassure them that you are still there for support (emotional and practical) and then gradually back off. If they simply like their comforts provided for them, then lay down some ground rules – share the chores including the cooking, charge rent if practical and learn to say 'no.'

EFFECT ON YOU

The National Housing Federation surveyed parents who had grown up children living at home. 23% percent reported that it caused them stress, 18% said it had triggered family arguments and 8% reported that it caused them to go into debt. It doesn't surprise me, mainly because I am still bailing out my twenty something daughters. The reason? Austerity has affected young people more than anyone. They are earning less (if they're lucky enough to have a job), prices are rocketing - including energy bills and council tax as well as rent - and the age for being able to get a deposit on a flat is rising year on year. Many of us imagined our children would go onto further education or go straight into a job and would swiftly fall off the parental pay role. In many families, this just hasn't happened and parents have had to use any savings they have or even downsize their property to support their twenty something children. It's the unexpected element which causes unrest while the family adjust to a new reality. We weren't really expecting it to turn out like this and neither were they.

One cause of stress is your son or daughter coming home and slipping straight into dependent child mode. The other cause of stress is a parent (so often the mother) slipping back into mummy mode. This can be put right once you recognise the symptoms, which are:

1. You catch yourself tucking your thirty year old up in bed and wondering where his teddy is.
2. Your son or daughter uses expressions such as 'it's not fair,' 'you love my sister more than me' and 'I hate broccoli, I told you.'
3. You think he or she should be wearing a vest now it's turned chilly.
4. Your child helps herself to all the best wine, your make up

and deluxe bathroom goods, borrows your clothes and then says 'everyone else is allowed to...'

5. You wait up for your 'child' to get in and then ask where she's been.
6. You read number five and wonder what's wrong with that.
7. Your child reads number five and wonders what's wrong with that.
8. You pick up clothes and towels and collect the dirty mugs. And say to yourself that while you're doing the washing/ironing, you might as well do hers.
9. She expects you to do all in number eight and get a meal on the table at a time suitable for her.
10. You think about going to the job interview with her. Or at least waiting outside. And you definitely print off the route/train times and put out clean clothes for her.

If your child has returned after university, then there will be a period of adjustment. You CAN'T just pick up from where you left off. She will have changed in ways you may not even realise. For one thing, she will have been cooking and cleaning (using the word cleaning loosely) for herself and both of you should expect this to continue. She will be three years older and a lot more mature and independent (hopefully). And she will have had to sort crises out FOR HERSELF. She won't be used to someone wanting to know where she is or what time she wants food. And you will have got used to having the house to yourself or just with you and your partner. There's been no one to question your taste in music, clothes or décor for some time. There's been no offspring to consider in your daily routine. You may suddenly feel less comfortable about smoking in the lounge/dancing to Billy Joel in the kitchen/ having sex on a Sunday afternoon. Give it time and look at all the positive things. After all, you cried nonstop for three weeks when she left.

EFFECT ON YOUR CHILD

Remember, just as you didn't expect your child to come back home to live, neither did she. This wasn't the plan, so there is a danger of resentment from your son or daughter when you are perhaps expecting gratitude. Your child may well be feeling very frustrated at not stepping into the high flying career university promised, or getting that promotion which would mean that renting a flat would be possible. She has to adjust to living with your rules and she may feel she's taken a step backwards. Her old pony pictures and photos of Take That in her room now seem strangely out of place and remind her that it's children who live at home with their parents, not adults. She may have friends who have been able to fly the nest and this can add to her frustration. So, show some understanding as to why she hasn't rushed home with open arms and hoping to stay until she's at least forty two.

1. Acknowledge that this wasn't plan A.
2. Talk about the advantages, financial and otherwise.
3. Tell her to let you know if you sink back into mummy mode (and you will let her know about kiddie mode.)
4. Tell her that she can stay as long as she wants, that it's her home too but also say that when the time's right, you'll assist in every practical way to help her move on.
5. Refrain from measuring her against the wall again.
6. Respect her privacy. It may have been acceptable to go into her room when she was nine but not at twenty nine.
7. 'But you always used to...' may not be the most helpful phrase.
8. Enjoy the unexpected parent-child times. She'll be off again one day so show her that you enjoy her company and make the most of the opportunity.
9. Have some weekends away with your partner or friends or on your own. Your son/daughter may like the house to

herself/himself occasionally. So might you, so encourage her to do the same every now and then.

10. She may find it awkward having friends round. Or she may not and have them round all the time. Late. Discuss it. Maybe you go to a club one day a week and you could encourage that to be her friends' night in.

11. Keep talking, keep adjusting until you all feel comfortable.

HOW TO MAKE IT WORK

1. Focus on all that's positive about having your adult child at home. This will be individual to you but may include having time together, sharing the cooking, having someone to give you a lift when you want to drink a bottle of wine somewhere, sharing clothes.

2. Don't let resentments fester. Maybe you find yourself screaming internally every time you find a dirty mug. Discuss it. Say how you feel.

3. Don't sweat the small stuff. Is the dirty mug that important? Why not ask her to go round and clear them up, rather than doing it yourself while simultaneously muttering remarks about mould, penicillin and deathly fungus under your breath.

4. Give it time.

5. Respect each other's privacy.

6. Let go. I can't say this enough. Let go, let go, let go. Two simple words (or six in my case) which say so much. Of course you want to pass on endless advice to your children, however old they are. You can SEE exactly where they're going wrong. You just KNOW that he isn't the right partner for her. You made the same mistake yourself so why not just TELL her. By all means, chat about these things but you're going to have to let her make her own mistakes. Ask if she wants your advice or wants to talk about it. If she doesn't,

just be there with the tissues when it all hits the fan.

7. Remember, if all had gone according to plan, she would have left home and be busy making all life's little mistakes we eventually learn from. So let go. See, I've said it again.

8. Don't keep reminding your child that it's your house, that you pay the bills and the rent/mortgage. After all, she would love to be paying a mortgage. It really is tougher out there for the next generation.

9. Try and eat together at least once a week.

10. Enjoy it. It won't last.

So far we have discussed a rather-fuller-than-expected nest but when your child finally leaves and you finally stop crying, you may well find yourself with a severe case of empty nest syndrome. She's flown away and your role will change almost overnight.

HOW TO HELP

1. Prepare the way. Your son or daughter needs to be able to cook, pay bills and generally take responsibility for his/her life. This is going to be far harder if you've always done everything for them. Start backing off early. Pass more decisions and responsibility on to them and teach them to cook. Do all of this WELL IN ADVANCE.

2. Don't be clingy. Some parents panic at the last minute and keep saying 'you can always change your mind,' 'I expect you'll come home a lot' and 'you will ring me twice a day, won't you.'

3. Let go. I may be writing those two words again.

4. Help with the actual moving. Make lists of items they need – they haven't done this before and may forget obvious essentials like loo paper, spare bedding and washing powder.

5. Be there afterwards. At the end of your phone if they need you, not sitting on their doorstep crying.

HOW TO SURVIVE

1. Start by congratulating yourself. You have bought up your child and she has not only survived but has the confidence to step out on her own. Job done.

2. Remind yourself that you haven't stopped being her mother just because she's not sleeping under your roof. But YOUR RELATIONSHIP WILL CHANGE. Of course it will, you can't possible have the same relationship as when she was five and you held her hand to cross the road. (If you are still holding her hand to cross the road, you have some serious thinking to do.) The relationship will be more one of friendship but with an added part time mentoring role. And I mean part time. You are there to advise IF SHE WANTS YOU TO. But you are now there primarily so you can enjoy each other's company. Sounds good to me.

3. This will be harder for mothers who have already given up work. But even so, it will leave a gap in your life. Fill that gap. Look on it as an opportunity to start that new hobby, change your job, do something you've always meant to do such as travel. Enjoy the new freedom.

4. Don't continue to parent. This doesn't mean you won't be on hand for practical help, emotional support and advice. But you don't need to phone every evening to make sure she's in, you don't need to go round and clean her flat and leave food parcels, and you don't need to panic if she hasn't texted you in the last hour.

5. Don't expect too much. You might think it would be great if she came home every Sunday for lunch. But she might not. Reach a compromise and remember that she has her own life to lead.

6. Don't try and move her on to the next stage in her life. You may want her to have a partner and produce some grandchildren for you. THAT IS HER DECISION and

nothing to do with you.

7. Do meet on neutral ground from time to time. If you go to her new abode, she may sense you looking at the pile of washing up and if she comes home to you, you may both slip into old patterns. Meet for coffee, go for a drink or a spa day, share your mutual interests whether that's going to the art gallery, theatre, cinema or pottery club. Like friends do.

8. Accept that you will go through a period of mourning. You may feel a sense of grief as you have lost a role. Accept support from family and friends and don't let anyone say 'snap out of it.' Why should you? Well, I suppose you should eventually – if you're still crying ten years later, you may need help. You will go in and out of this mourning phase – so just let it be and at the same time, move on.

9. DON'T be secretly pleased if they're unhappy. Or if they miss home.

10. DO be extra nice to yourself. You have your bathroom back so indulge in some luxury bath oils. You have a bit of extra time, so spend it on yourself.

UNIVERSITY CHALLENGE

This is a wonderful way of leaving home as it is gradual. Your offspring will be home in the holidays and may even be able to have a couple of long weekends home during the term time. The permanent leaving of home won't take place until after graduating (and as discussed earlier, this may be well after graduating.) It's still a life changing rite of passage and it would be odd if you both didn't feel a little nervous. Let's have a list to help you….

1. Don't be a helicopter parent. I see a boutique hotel has just sprung up right near the halls of residence at Sheffield University. Tempted to stay there every weekend? Don't.

Tempted to go down and clean up while she's at a lecture? Of course you are but PLEASE resist. Helicopter parenting has got so bad that some parents even go into the actual interview for Uni (or a job) with their son/daughter. If you do give your child a lift to the interview, keep well out of the way. Do not pace up and down in the corridor outside – you shouldn't even be in the building. Or the grounds.

2. You will be thinking drugs, drop outs, drunken nights walking home alone, forgetting to get up for three weeks and all the other possible things that can go wrong. You could drive yourself NUTS with worst case scenarios, so don't. All right, you can't stop yourself but at least try and be logical. Your child has got this far without falling to all the demons you are imagining, and if there's been some dabbling, it must have been just that – SHE'S GOT INTO UNI. And you don't do that if you're addicted to everything and you never showed up at school. Have the conversation but keep it brief. And just ensure they know where the support and counselling is at the Uni. All Unis have support for students who get into difficulty and yes, they do notice if a student is not turning up to any tutorials.

3. Think about how and when you communicate. And how often. Your child won't appreciate a long phone call when she's out with her new mates. Once she has her schedule, you can talk about when's a good time to chat. Not every day but maybe once a week. Twice a week if you really insist, at least to start with. Texts are much better. They are less intrusive and you are less likely to be over anxious in your tone. But if she doesn't answer within sixty seconds, don't then imagine she must be at the bottom of the lake and then phone just to check. She will reply. Eventually. Don't panic if she doesn't tell you much. This is her chance to be independent so she really won't want to report back every detail of her life in

hourly texts. As a general rule, no news is good news. She is more likely to be phoning when she needs assistance.

4. Don't be a check list Mum. No need to ask her if she's washed her bedding, if she's eating properly and is getting her essays in on time. It's up to her now. Your job is to offer support when needed and let her get on with it.

5. There will be times when things don't go according to plan. Maybe she's having trouble settling in, is doubting her choice of course or is missing her home or her home town. Your job is to listen, sympathise and guide her into sorting it out. FOR HERSELF. Don't drive straight down and sort it out for her. Don't be a rescuer – the main purpose of leaving home is to become independent and you can't do that with a Mum who just sorts it all out for you. So if she has money concerns (she will have) then help her with a budget, don't bail her out every time.

If you want your child to have a positive experience leaving home, then you need to be positive too. It's not going to help if you go round listing all the things that can possibly go wrong. It won't help if she senses your anxiety, especially if your anxiety is unfounded and possibly more to do with your loss than anything else. I still remember taking my eldest daughter to Bristol and her bottom lip quivering as we unloaded her things from the car. Then I noticed other girls in her hall looking equally shell shocked. I went out, bought a couple of bottles of wine and told her to invite everyone into a room for a drink. I didn't do it for her and I wondered if she'd have the courage. I could only advise and the rest was up to her. She did, and she is still friends with that group of girls several years later. A good bit of parenting. Nice to know I can get it right every now and then.

My friend's youngest daughter left home to begin a textiles course and she moved in with her boyfriend at the same time. Her boyfriend was a lovely young man, very bright and very caring. Even so, both her parents were fairly certain this would end in tears. However, this was not their decision to make and they duly moved them in and left to see what would happen. Later, it did end in tears and the girl asked her boyfriend to move out (nothing he'd done wrong, just an inevitable end). My friend ended up paying his share of the rent while she finished her course. She knew that this was rescuing her, which I had advised against, but I suspect I would have done the same thing. In the end it was a matter of damage limitation. It was a life's lesson, but rather an expensive one. If I'm honest, I do think I too have been a bit of a rescuer as a parent but I did eventually learn to step back. It's not just our children who need to learn from mistakes. And I'm still learning.

MONEY ISSUES

This will be a big learning curve for all children leaving home. I really do wish they would teach money management in schools as it is such an important life skill and one we so often learn the hard way. According to the CSFI (centre for the study of financial innovation) 64% of young people have had no formal financial education. To be honest, I would have put it higher than that. So, until finance is taught at school as a life skill, we have a role to play as parents.

One problem, if it is indeed a problem, is that according to research 80-85% of young people are very optimistic about their future, more than older generations. I'm sure that's true – when you are young, you believe you are indestructible and that rules of health and safety don't really apply to you. You drive fast, drink too much, take risks. Your judgements are impaired by all those hormones. And that's why the following came out of the research:

1. Many young people don't consider student debt to be a debt

at all.

2. Four in ten young earners who contribute to a pension don't know what sort of pension it is.

3. 41% estimate that they will buy their first house in their twenties (the reality is that it will be at least their late thirties, if at all.)

The reality is, there is high youth unemployment and that since 2007, the number of graduates doing so called menial jobs (bar work, cleaning) has doubled. Of course not all young people are unrealistic or even optimistic and there are many who see no hope at all. But for those who do have an income or are trying to manage their student loan, the chances are they will have poor money management skills.

Without resorting to phrases like 'in the good old days,' I can't help wonder if it was a whole lot easier when we had pay packets with actual money in. Or at least when we were a predominantly cash and cheque society. It's so easy to wield a card without relating it to actual money. Both my daughters have been taken by surprise when they have had a card refused because they had exceeded their overdraft limit. And what were the banks doing giving them overdrafts in the first place? One when she was just embarking on her acting career, before she even had her first job, and the other straight out of Uni.

Luckily both daughters are earning and seem to be getting through life well, with just the occasional dip into the bank of mum and dad (yes, I know we shouldn't but we're weak). I did, however, give them financial advice as did their father. I can't claim it had a great effect, they still see money management as spending until you run out and don't worry about tomorrow. But despite my limited success, here is my advice to them:

1. Deal in cash. Take out your money for the week and then you

can see what you have left. Or at least check your balance frequently.

2. When you have earned a bit more, put it to one side (preferably earning interest) until an emergency. Yes, one day your phone or laptop will break or you will need to take a trip somewhere so be prepared.

3. Write down everything you spend. When you see exactly what you spend each month on takeaway coffees, then you will probably end up using a flask.

4. Look for bargains in the supermarket. Shop late when they are selling things off.

5. DON'T have a credit card until you are earning enough to warrant it. And when you do, pay it off as soon as possible.

All right, there are those who will give better advice, but that was what I came up with. I felt sorry for them, particularly when they were students. It is just so easy to borrow money, have an overdraft and take as many credit cards as you care to have. It shouldn't be that way but it is. There is also a culture of debt among the young where it seems perfectly acceptable to run up as much debt as you can muster.

The reason for going off on this financial tangent is to point out that as older women with older children, we have a role to play in guiding them in all matters financial, because the chances are they'll be rubbish at it. Not that it's easy but it seems to be one of the biggest challenges they face. In some ways we are passing down the benefit of our experience but in other ways, our experience was very different. I remember as a student being called into the back of the bank to be 'told off' because I'd gone overdrawn. This, of course, was pre student loans but that's a whole new debate we don't have time to discuss here. Except to acknowledge that the financial pressures on the next generation down are greater than ever. So if you have any wisdom to impart, then go on and impart. Just don't expect total compliance with your ideas. Like everything else, there will be a lot of learning from their own mistakes.

It's perhaps ironic, that just at the time you will be trying to help your children adjust to being responsible for their own finances, you may have some financial adjustments of your own to make as you retire or prepare for retirement. There are plenty of parents wanting to retire, ready to retire and financially secure enough to retire but they are waiting for the 'children' to be more financially stable. A personal choice of course, but do bear in mind that they may never be completely financially stable. Are you going to hang on at work forever?

SOMEONE ELSE IN THE NEST

So, your last child leaves home, you have a tearful and sleepless night and then you come down to breakfast in the morning to something you haven't heard for a while – silence. No sound of thumping music and cries of 'have you seen my jumper?' All is strangely quiet and serene but then you notice someone opposite you at the breakfast table. You know the face and eventually you put a name to him (or her). It's your partner. The one you set up home with but looking a little more jaded now.

It's likely that your children have been the focus of your life for many years. First they were babies keeping you up at night, then they were toddlers keeping you up at night and after a short reprieve, they turned into teenagers keeping you up at night. You love them more than anything but it would be odd if you hadn't torn at least one hair out along the way. And all your decisions would have been made with the thought of how it might affect the children at the back of your mind. In fact, most of your decisions were ABOUT the children. Your life will have been your children in the centre with you are your partner frantically running round the outside, looking in. The chances are you haven't looked at your partner for years. If things have been really child focused, you may not remember his name. You may feel you know your child's teacher more intimately and you will have certainly forgotten the dim and distant past when your partner was just that – your partner and not the children's parent or step-parent.

Then one day, there he (or she) is. The children have flown the nest and you've forgotten what to do. You talk about what your offspring might be doing and when all possibilities have been exhausted, you realise that you are now both just redundant parents without a portfolio. Surely there's more to you than that. Of course, you are only really in waiting until the first distress call comes through but in the mean time, you can be a couple. A proper couple who only have eyes for each other. The problem is, you've forgotten how. And you might have forgotten just who that person opposite you at the breakfast table really is. Or maybe you've just been reminded that the children were actually the only thing you had in common which might not leave you with much of a future.

More couples in their fifties are getting divorced than ever before in what I call the twenty seven year mass itch. It seems to coincide with the children flying the nest and in some instances, couples will have stayed together for the children's sake and now they've gone, so is the reason for being an item. Other couples will need to re-discover each other and re-negotiate their relationship. It's all change, one way or another.

Yes, there's some huge readjustment to be made even for the happiest of couples and with the children gone, it will all look very different. You may not like the face across the breakfast table any more, (maybe you haven't for a while), or the spark may have gone out of your relationship and you hadn't noticed because you'd been too busy helping your child write endless application forms and treating acne. It's the end of an era and you may see a bleak future ahead of retirement, gardening and having your partner at home twenty four hours a day. You may even find you have differing ideas about your future. It's a minefield. I don't suppose there are many couples who shout hooray as they wave their child off, decide to have rampant sex in every room in the house and take up new joint hobbies so they can spend every spare minute together in post children rapture.

A personal note – I missed my children so much, that it never occurred to me that John missed them too. We could have talked about that but we didn't. I had this nagging feeling that the best years we'd spent together were behind us and I did wonder whether it was therefore worth carrying on. I looked back with fondness but looked ahead with fear and confusion. Then I realised I didn't need to look ahead, I just needed to think about now. And we needed to move into this new era of our life gradually. And just as it took some adjusting to having children and being a family for the first time, so it would take some adjusting to being parents from a distance. So we took our time and we moved onto our new era together. However, we did see several marriages of our contemporaries crumble and every time that happened, I felt quite shaken. It was so easy. You didn't have the children to think of (although that's not quite true – children of ALL ages are affected by parental divorce and separation) and I could see how some couples might rush into a split out of a sort of blind panic.

If you did stay together for the children and you've been waiting for this day, then go ahead. Never a good idea to stay together because it's the easy option. But if you want to carry on but are struggling, then think about the following:-

1. It takes time to adjust to any change.
2. You will need to acknowledge how you feel about waving goodbye to the last to leave home. And it's not just a mother's

prerogative – missing them is something you share.

3. Just as you had to compromise and negotiate how to be parents as you were bringing them up, you will need to negotiate with your partner how to help when you get that frantic phone call (usually about money.) It's no good one of you bailing them out, while the other is determined they learn the hard way. In our case, we bailed them out rather too readily and on more than one occasion found they had approached us separately for a 'loan'. (NB a loan to your children rarely gets paid back. Accept and move on.)

4. It's worth re-visiting why you set up home together in the first place. It's that feeling of love and total commitment that you're looking to re-ignite. It won't ever be exactly the same but it's what your relationship is based on.

5. Talk about the advantages of being back on your own. And act on them. You have more freedom, you don't have to consider the children when you choose a holiday location, you can wear what you like without a teenager saying 'are you going out in that?' You can watch what you like on TV. And much more.

6. Have date nights. It's easy to slip into 'Now she's gone, I'll clean out the garage,' mode.

7. I love it when I see much older couples sitting on deckchairs and holding hands. You can tell they've lived a shared life and are going to see it out together. If that's what you want, it's worth working at it.

8. But if it's not what you want, then say so. Don't spend the last years of your life hating each other. You really don't have to.

9. Don't get in a rut. It gets easier to get in a rut as you get older. Your children will have kept you young. Your children will have encouraged you to do new things. Just because they don't live under your roof, it doesn't mean you have to suddenly age and do the same thing every day. Be even more

171

adventurous, daring and outrageous.

10. You may decide that the next stage is being a grandparent. BUT THAT'S NOT UP TO YOU. So, DON'T try and push your child's relationship into that stage. If you catch yourself saying, 'why don't you have a one night stand and see what the result is' you've got far too desperate. And desperate for something that's not your decision.

BEING GRANDPARENTS

Perhaps this warrants a whole chapter to itself – it certainly does seem to be a big topic. But at the time of writing, we don't have the sound of grandchildren's feet pattering about, so I don't have the experience to offer much in the way of advice or wisdom on the matter. So I'll condense it.

1. Don't interfere when the parents choose the name of your first grandchild. Unless they choose IKEA. Or COWELL.
2. Don't interfere with anything after the baby is born. Unless the parents do anything dangerous. Or embarrassing.
3. Enjoy it all.

That's all you need to know.

BEING IN YOUR OWN NEST (RETIREMENT)

Of course your nest will eventually get filled by you. But the whole nature of retirement is changing. Firstly, the government have introduced laws which mean you don't have to retire at a particular time and can stay on for as long as you want or are able to (with a few notable exceptions). This is inevitable if you think about it. Sixty and seventy year olds are fitter than ever, there will be more older people out there needed in their jobs and many of us have seen our pension prospects diminished. Why would we not work if we are fit and want to carry on having the money to enjoy our lives?

There may be some barriers - Mariella Frostrup recently

claimed that her workload halved as soon as she reached fifty. However, the law is on our side for those of us already employed and hoping to stay on. For those who may be returning to work, the good news is that Ros Altmann, the business champion for older workers, has proposed that people over fifty be offered internships to begin new careers. There has already been interest by some heavyweight companies and Ros is hoping to persuade the government that older internees are offered the same sort of job subsidies that young people receive. This may all then help change the culture so that it has a knock on effect for the self employed over fifties, including those in the public eye such as Mariella, who have seen their workload go down.

Some of you, of course, may welcome a cut down and the government are also encouraging companies to recognise the benefits of a gradual retirement. The days of being presented with a watch on your sixtieth birthday and going home to realise a watch is the last thing you need any more, are long gone. You may well feel far too young to give up work at sixty six but you may be in a position to cut your hours, then or much earlier. Retirement is gradually turning into a PROCESS rather than an EVENT and middle-aged and older women are really welcoming this change. So, you may choose to go back into the nest or may just want to hop out from time to time. More choices can only be good for everyone.

TWELVE: THE 'M' WORD

You can't really have a book with the sub title of 'How To Be An Older Woman' without having a discussion about the menopause. In fact, many of you may have decided to read this book imagining that's what it would be all about. It's not, but it has been allocated its own chapter so it's up there with sex and feminism. There will be better books and websites than this to give you the sort of medical advice you might want but this is a chance to think about what it all means. And how we might want to change attitudes towards it.

The most important thing to hang on to is that THE MENOPAUSE IS NORMAL. It's not some rare disease, it certainly isn't (or shouldn't be) an embarrassing one. It's normal. It's what all women go through. If you're ninety years old, still having periods and still worrying about getting pregnant then you are the unusual one, not the rest of us. So just as puberty is a normal stage of development, then so is the menopause. All right pubescent girls might not SEEM normal, but they are. If you count storming out of the house and hiding round the back of Dorothy Perkins sulking with a spotty face and an attitude normal.

WHAT IS IT?

Quite simply, it's the closing down of the egg factory. Your ovaries stop churning out an egg every month, your periods stop and your child producing days are over. It's gradual and is caused by the natural change in balance of the body's sex organs. Your oestrogen goes down a bit, basically. Sounds straight forward. And yet, the word menopause seems more loaded than that, brings up all sorts of thoughts, images and emotions with it. Yes, it's a minefield.

TALKING ABOUT IT

As a rule, we don't seem to like talking about it. Have you ever found yourself talking about the menopause in the back bar in between a conversation about the football league and a debate about Miley Cyrus? I thought not. It's just so embarrassing. Really? We're happy to talk all things sex, we relish a conversation about the sordid affairs of some celebrity, we show each other piercings and tattoos in the most intimate places. But the menopause? Oh no, too embarrassing. Try bringing up the details of your menopause in conversation and unless you're talking about it to another menopausal woman, you might find your listener changing the subject rather swiftly. It's probably because they think you might mention periods. Shocking. However, things are changing and young girls talk about periods more readily than we did. In my day, it was the curse, now girls call it their friend. A tad too far maybe, but still, it's out there on display. Or nearly.

Perhaps when the next generation get to their menopause, they will make another friend and have menopausal discussions in the pub as a matter of course, with the barman joining in with an anecdote about how he's supporting his wife through it (as he puts a bottle of gin in his rucksack.) But right now, it's still a bit of an uncomfortable topic. Online forums may help to change all that. It might be that it's easier to start by commenting as an anonymous hot-flusher so that soon you'll be able to shout 'vaginal dryness' out loud in Sainsbury's. But the most important thing is to TALK ABOUT IT. I don't mean non-stop like a monologue you call out as you walk along the street (though feel free, if it helps). I mean talk to friends going through the same stage as you, so that you can share experiences and tips, talk to your partner so he understands why you've just emptied the water from the flower vase all over your head, and talk about it to everyone and anyone so that we keep moving away from the days when the menopause was whispered about behind cupped hands. We no longer need to say 'Auntie Flo has left the building', 'I've got a new weather system,' or 'The maternity suite is closed for business.' We can say MENOPAUSE as loudly as we like. No, I don't much like the word either. Like menstruation - that's a horrid word too. All medical, like a nasty tropical disease. And do these words really have to begin with men? I'd like a new word that sounds more, well, friendly. But not some sort of euphemism like Auntie Flo. It's sometimes called the change of life which is OK, but sounds a bit like you're going to move to Bournemouth and buy a café. How about the monthlygone or the hooraytime. Something more fun and positive anyway. But for now it's menopause and all we can do is articulate the word in a fun and positive tone – Menopause, trala!

Because we haven't talked about it much in the past (though things are beginning to change), there are a number of myths out there. Men in particular are a bit woolly about the whole thing so let's dispel a few of those myths first.

MENOPAUSAL MYTHS

1. The menopause is a medical condition that requires treatment.

No. Most women go through the menopause with a few symptoms but they don't feel ill. There's no need to rush off to the doctor at the first flush, demanding HRT, a bottle of vodka and a short rest in hospital. It's a normal stage. Some women might need some help with symptoms if they are affected badly but these tend to be the minority. However, if you are one of those struggling with the symptoms do talk to your doctor. Some women swear by HRT. And a few women might need something to help them deal with temporary heavy periods.

2. Menopause is the first step on the road to death.

You are closer to death as you get older. The menopause doesn't fast track you. Women are still living longer than men on average and they don't experience the menopause (whatever they tell you).

3. You will be in the depths of despair.

The menopause doesn't cause depression. It coincides with a time of your life when there are other changes such as children flying the nest and this may be the cause of feeling down. Yes, there are hormone changes and this can lead to mood swings. But not depression, as such.

4. Nothing going on between the sheets.

See the sex chapter. You may need a lubricant. You may need your partner to boost your confidence. You may temporarily lose a bit of libido. But no need to stop.

5. Nothing going on between the ears.

The menopause does not leave you standing in the kitchen wondering why you even went in there. It does not mean you start chatting to your neighbour you've known for ten years and call her Betty when she's called Camilla. And it doesn't mean you find yourself pacing the supermarket car park searching for your parked car. Age does that. Not the menopause.

6. You will begin to look older

Only because you are older.

7. You can never be more than fifty metres from the toilet.

The menopause doesn't cause incontinence. It can happen as you get older but it is not a symptom of the menopause.

8. You will be hard of hearing, short sighted and with creaking bones.

Your body is getting older and there may be some wear and tear. No more for women than for men.

9. As soon as you miss a period, you don't have to worry about pregnancy.

You need to wait a year after your periods stop before you are safe (two years if you have an early menopause). Unless you want a little brother for your teenage children. A toddler, a couple of teenagers and a menopausal woman make an interesting combination. There might be a dad in that list, but he's probably hiding in the attic.

10. You have to dress in purple and run your stick along the railings.

That's just a poem. Mind you, it has some top ideas in it.

11. You will be completely out of date and stop watching Top of the Pops.

Top of the Pops? (Replace that thought with whatever the current music programmes are.) You can be as up to date as you like. The menopause won't stop you. In fact, I recommend keeping a tab on what's going on now. Menopausal women are not a separate species stuck in Beatle-land, talking about 'new-fangled' things and wondering what happened to all the telephone boxes.

WHEN DOES IT HAPPEN?

The average age for reaching the menopause is fifty one and a half. Some authorities say fifty one (usually the American ones) and some say fifty two. So I'm saying fifty one and a half. That's just an average of course and like starting your periods, the exact age varies. There have been some women in their late fifties who have suddenly fallen pregnant quite naturally and for some women it's all over far sooner. If you reach the menopause before the age of forty five, then it's known as an early menopause. If you are under forty, then it's a premature menopause and you will almost certainly find yourself at the GP to get this confirmed with a blood test.

There is a fairly strong hereditary factor – if your mother had an early or late onset, you are likely to as well. My mother was bang on time. I remember it well because she was particularly hit by mood swings. To be fair, she always had mood swings but at last she had something to blame them on.

Ethnicity has an effect, with Chinese and Japanese a little later than white women. Smokers tend to have an earlier menopause and obviously if you have had ovarian surgery this may trigger an early menopause. If you have your ovaries removed completely then you'll be thrown straight into it. No warm up, no dress rehearsal, just the real thing and as sudden as when One Direction arrived. Quite similar, I suppose. One minute all was well with the world, and the next minute, everything's changed. And to start with you're going to be wishing you were back in the days of the Beatles. Then you get used to it and think there may be some advantages to Harry Styles. Obviously, you get medical advice at the time of your op and you are likely to be given HRT.

If you only have a hysterectomy and they leave your ovaries behind, you'll be better off. They haven't left them in as part of the NHS cuts but because it prevents you being thrown into that sudden menopause. And the menopause is generally thought to be better if it creeps up slowly behind you. Like age itself. There is some evidence that your menopause may come slightly earlier as a result of your hysterectomy but not hugely. I had a hysterectomy and never felt better in the weeks afterwards. My unmanageably heavy periods were gone and I felt like a new woman. I think I may have hit the menopause now but to be honest symptoms are few. And as my periods have stopped as a result of my operation, it's hard to say what's going on. Many women, like me, report very little in the way of symptoms and the symptoms they have are manageable. In that way, it's much the same as puberty. I had one daughter who was mildly moody and seemed to sail through it all and the other who swung from one extreme mood to another in a way that frightened us all. One minute she was making me a cup of tea and being the perfect daughter and the next minute she was putting a brick though the window. To be fair to her, she only did that once and she was as surprised as we were (and she's lovely now), but it's a good example of how hormone changes affect everyone differently. A quick run through the symptoms with some possible solutions but for further help, there are numerous websites.

SYMPTOMS

1.Hot flushes.

Americans call these hot flashes, which sounds like a man exposing himself in August. These can last just a few moments or ten minutes. You suddenly feel very hot, may go a bit red and may sweat. HRT helps if they are unbearable but do take practical measures such as carrying a hand held fan about with you in your handbag. Also, wear layers so that you can whip a cardie off quickly in an emergency. Some women find it embarrassing, aware that they look a bit hot and sweaty. Probably best just to explain. This will also, hopefully, result in some sympathy in the office, rather than annoyance, when you fling open all the windows in December. Don't forget, humour can help get everyone on board. So find your own quirky phrase – I'm just taking a personal trip to the tropics, or I'm having my own private climate change. This is not to encourage euphemisms to avoid talking about it properly, but humour invites everyone in to the conversation. Being able to laugh at yourself will help you and doesn't have to mean you're trivialising it.

2. Night sweats.

Who needs global warming with all this going on? Your partner will have to agree to the window open. Cold? He can wear thicker pyjamas. Cotton sheets will be needed and two single duvets on a double bed works well so you can fling your own off. For this and for hot flushes, there may be triggers. Yes, obviously the menopause IS the trigger, but there are certain foods which may make it worse for you. Common culprits are caffeine, alcohol (sorry) and spicy foods. Some women have even reported cheese as a trigger. Keep a diary of when the flushes occur and the night sweats (night, obviously) and your diet. There may even be emotional triggers. As with everything ever listed on any health and well being site ever, exercise is recommended. It seems to be a cure all activity which is absolutely free. All you have to do is step outside your door and start jogging. Or brisk walking. Or at least park your car down the road a bit and stroll a few metres into work.

3. Vaginal Dryness.

Get a lubricant.

4. Mood Swings.

Sometimes hormonal changes can cause mood swings. Acknowledge this, both to yourself and others. Feel like killing your husband? It may not be his fault, it may be a mood swing, in which case explain how you feel to him. Tell him you are doing your best to control it. And apologise if an apology is due, while handing him a leaflet about menopausal mood swings. Still feel like killing your husband and can list several perfectly legitimate reasons why? That might not be your hormones so address the problems. But don't kill him, you'll be banged up with a lot of other hormonal women. Ways to cope – I can't recommend meditation enough. A short daily meditation will change your life. If you don't know how to start – it couldn't be simpler so a book may help or a local class. But DO IT – it's the best mood leveller known. If you know your mood is shaky and it is practical to do so, BE ON YOUR OWN. Just for a while. Go for a walk, have a long bath, meditate or listen to some uplifting music. Moods can be changed, or at least bettered and it's a matter of finding what works for you. I have written out all my favourite poems in one handy note book. And I have a list of all my favourite mood-changing music tracks on Spotify. And if none of that works, I throw crockery. Luckily for anyone in my firing line, poetry and music and especially meditation really do work.

5. Sleep problems.

Sometimes this is linked to being woken with night sweats, sometimes it's linked to anxiety and sometimes it's linked to your bladder needing to be emptied more often. Again, be mindful of caffeine and alcohol and don't exercise late in the day. Have a wind down time with a bath and a book and try and empty your mind of all problems. One way of doing this is to write down what's going round and round in your mind in a notebook. This reinforces the fact that you will deal with it tomorrow and there is nothing further you can do that day. If necessary, do your version of counting sheep – a mundane series of thoughts to get all stimulating ideas out of your mind. Think of names of poets beginning with each letter of the alphabet, for example. This is particularly good for getting back to sleep after a disruption. And try and go to bed at a similar time each night.

6. Period Problems.

Rarely do your periods just stop. Last one on 27th November and you never have another one. Much more likely that they will be less frequent and a bit more spasmodic. Imagine if you don't quite know when your in-laws are going to turn up, or you're expecting them on the weekend of the 30th, only to find they turn up a week early. Or they don't bother turning up at all. And you don't quite know what they're going to bring with them but there's a good chance they'll turn up with way too much stuff. That's what it's like. So you have to be prepared all the time. And just when you think you've got rid of your unwelcome guest for good, here she is again.

7. Weight gain.

Post menopausal women tend to thicken up round the waist a bit. But this is a tendency not a rule. Some of you will happily accept your body shape, others might want to do a lot of sit ups and watch their diet. Your choice. Not anyone else's choice, not society's choice, but yours.

8. All of the above and so much more.

For some, the menopause gets a bit more unruly. This will be for the minority but if it's you, then you really do need some extra help. So do visit your GP and she or he will talk you through the options including HRT. There are alternatives as well including herbal remedies so look them up and see what's out there. As promised, I am not going into medical details here but you don't, these days, have to put up with total discomfort and overwhelming symptoms. Grin and bear it, my mother used to say about such things. Why?

AND ON THE PLUS SIDE...

Menopausal women get a bit of a bad press. As do older women in general, as we know. There is so much that is positive about getting through the menopause and yet we tend to focus on all that's wrong with it. You say the word menopause to some and they immediately think of bad tempered women who are past their sell by date and could grow a small beard if they wanted. But for many women, it leads to a new lease of life. After all it's just a transition and when you get out the other side, you are not thrown into the reject pile or taken to the council tip like something that's clearly beyond recycling. You are not sat in a rocking chair in the corner with people bringing you cups of tea and a garibaldi. You are still out there, living your life to the full. And if you are not, re-read this book and ask yourself what's stopping you.

Time to celebrate what the menopause means to you and all that's wonderful about it. Yes, wonderful.

1. You can have safe, free sex. No fear of pregnancy and you have all that experience. Share it with a younger lover if you're so inclined (and if it suits your situation). All the rage these days. This is the age of 'the bedroom ain't for sleeping in.'

2. Sexual freedom invariably spreads to the other areas of your life. This is the age where you really don't have to care what people think. You've had years of being self conscious, a life time of worrying if someone even glances at you. If not now,

when? So skip up the road in a onesie singing songs from the shows if you feel like it. This is the age of 'I'll do what the hell I like.'

3. No more periods. Enough said.

4. You are heading for retirement so what have you go to lose. Take risks at work, go for that promotion, apply for a new job or a whole new career. This is the age of 'why not?'

5. As with any transition in life, you will suddenly be aware that your time on this earth is limited. So you have a choice – start saving for your funeral and make sure all your affairs are in order or get on with that thing you always meant to try. You can do both but I know which I'd do first. So what was is you said you wished you'd done – write a book? Go on a TV panel show? Enter your painting for a competition? Run onto a football pitch naked? This is the age of 'regrets, I've had a few so I'll put them right, right now.'

6. This is often when women start to look outside their families. Mainly because the offspring have gone and you can't have any more. So what do you really care passionately about – women's rights? Local politics? The environment? Whatever it is, you have experience, often time, and a new found zest for life which will enable you to contribute to a cause close to your heart. This is the age of 'I'm going to change the world.'

7. Some women will finally realise they will never have a family. All right, you've known for some time. But now is the time to see if you want to get involved with children in some other way. A friend of mine has one grown up child – a gay son who has no interest in having children. So, not likely to be a granny then. But she's stepped in to help with the Rainbows and Brownies and loves it. Particularly impressive as she was thrown out of the guides herself. This is the age of enjoying kids which you can then give back when they start to get annoying.

8. You can take pride in having got this far intact. A bit battered and bruised maybe, but in one piece. And you can stand back and watch all the younger women make the same mistakes as you did. You might want to step in and help or offer advice. Or you might just want to be smug. This is the age of 'done that, got the T shirt.'

9. You can accept yourself as you are. A bit thicker round the waist maybe – so what? Can't find the car keys for the third time that day – so what – they are bound to be somewhere. Need stronger reading glasses so you can check if the instructions are in English. Or find the instructions. Or find the new item you need the instructions for? No problem – it's something else to laugh about in the pub. This is the age of 'if you can't laugh at yourself, who can you laugh at?'

10. You can look back and reminisce about when you were younger. But when you delve deeper, you will realise that it wasn't easy, it was often painfully hard and you didn't know what you were doing half the time. Chances are that as you get older, you accept your faults, you feel more comfortable in your skin and you are happier. And if that isn't true for you, then be aware that IT IS POSSIBLE.

The menopause needs re-branding. A new, positive name might help but then Snickers is still Marathon whichever way you look at it. What would help is a new image. Wear a T shirt – Menopausal and Proud. Or just think it to yourself. If life is really just a real version of a popular computer game, you've made it to the next level and you've collected a lot of points along the way. If life is just a reality show, congratulations – you're through to the next round. And don't wait to get near the end before you start to enjoy it. ENJOY EVERY MOMENT. Look how far we've come. Our mothers and grandmothers may have been content to wield the frying pan in an old apron and those slippers with the zip up the front. But menopausal women today are out there doing it. There are menopausal politicians, pop stars, board room members and others successful in their own fields. And we look at them and think of them as successful, influential women first and foremost. We don't look at them and think – 'I hope she's got her fan and her HRT pills in her bag or she's done for.'

It's time to celebrate the menopause, not be frightened of it. My mother often reminded me of when she told me all about periods. She may have been a bit graphic because apparently my response was – 'no thanks, I think I'll give them a miss.' She failed to explain that they would happen whether I wanted them to or not. Well the same goes for the menopause. It will happen so you might as well accept it and look on the bright side of it all. Maybe there should be a rite of passage. First hot flush? – Announce it on Facebook and invite all your friends round to crack open a bottle of gin. Missed a period? - go back to the first place you made love with your partner and do it all over again, but better. A year since your last period – do whatever you want. For the rest of your life.

THIRTEEN: LET'S GET POLITICAL

Feminism is political. It's about making sure it's an equal world and then maintaining that equal world. Ageism is political for the same reason. So we're all political in one way or another. But sometimes ranting in the pub or posting a comment on line doesn't seem enough. So we band together and rant in a bigger group or we comment on influential websites on mass. Now that feels a bit more political. But we also need representation where it counts. We need older women in positions of power so we can feed our views in to them and they can make a difference on our behalf. And we're getting there. Slowly. Very slowly.

A LITTLE BIT OF HISTORY

I have already indicated that although we have a way to go, we are making progress. Let's give this some context. Just over a hundred years ago, there were no female politicians in the Houses of Parliament. Not one. Maybe a woman scrubbing the floor and checking under the benches for sweet wrappers, but none of them actually sitting on the benches making decisions. Now nearly a quarter of MPs are women and one in five of those sitting in the House of Lords are women. So progress. But of course, if Parliament is there to represent the people, then it ought to look a bit more like the world it represents. With at least half the members women. That has to be the long term aim. And not too long term, either.

The first woman elected to Parliament was Countess Constance de Markievicz in 1918. Yes, I thought it was Nancy Astor as well. Seems the countess was in prison at the time so was unable to take up her seat for Sinn Fein but Nancy Astor managed to get her bum well and truly planted on a bench. There followed a mini surge after women got equal voting rights and so in 1929, there were 16 women. Now fast forward to 1997 the number of female MPs doubled from sixty to one hundred and twenty largely down to Labour's all female shortlist policy. Good news for democracy, rather spoilt by the fact that the new women MPs became known as Blair's Babes. Oh dear.

For a long time women remained on the back benches in the shadows. Then came Margaret Thatcher who famously said that she would not see a woman Prime Minister in her lifetime, then became one in 1979 and refused to budge from her post for eleven years and two hundred and nine days. That should have been a great time for women in politics but that's debatable and we will, indeed, debate it shortly. We had the first female leader of the House of Lords in 1981 and the first female speaker, Betty Boothroyd, in 1992. So we are on our way. However, it is not only important that we get more female representation in Parliament and lots of it, but that we have a high quality of women MPs and have women MPs who will make a difference to women's causes.

QUALITY AND QUANTITY

There has been a debate about women's shortlists since they became a popular proposition in the 1990s. The sex discrimination act has an amendment to allow all political parties to use all women shortlists if they choose, to ensure more female MPs are elected. It is labour who have really made use of this, leading to an increase in female politicians in 1997 in particular. The argument against them is that this is not true equality and that politicians should be elected on merit with no regards to what sex they are. It has also been suggested that all women shortlists would result in some sub standard women being elected and that would, in turn, give all female MPs a bad name. But these arguments are not nearly as compelling as the ones in favour of them.

1. High calibre female politicians have been elected as a result of all women shortlists. It was one such shortlist which gave

us our first female home secretary.

2. The house of commons needs to reflect our society and so we need more women. This needs a kick start, that's all. I believe the legislation that allows for the shortlists only lasts until 2030 by which time it is expected that they will not be needed.

3. We are making up for lost time. For too long there have been many, many all male shortlists.

4. Before all women shortlists, there was a percentage of the population who unconsciously thought of MPs as men, just as years ago if you said the word 'doctor' a male figure sprang to mind. All women shortlists bypass any unconscious pre-conception until such time as MPs are thought of as either male or female. And yes, we're getting there with that.

5. In an ideal world, women would have come to the forefront naturally but we know that in many walks of life including business and science, women need to be BETTER than their male counterparts to succeed.

In a similar vein, there has also been an ongoing debate about boardroom quotas where a percentage of the board must be female, again in order to kick start the necessary change and in light of the old boys' network which we know is still an influence. In this country, this is done on a voluntary basis but maybe we should look at countries like Norway who have made it law. Apparently, it's working there and everyone involved is happy about it so perhaps we should follow suit. I will leave the business women among you to debate that one. But in my opinion, we often need to take bold action to instigate change.

We can't talk about quality without mentioning Margaret Thatcher. Did she do anything for women? The short answer is 'No.' The long answer is 'Noooo!' Quite simply, Thatcher surrounded herself with men and did not believe in feminism (apparently) or helping the sisterhood. She said that women should rise up by their own merit and at that time men had all the merit. So we had slimy Cecil Parkinson rather than what should have been up-and-coming and reliable Lynda Chalker. With a wealthy husband and her own success, Thatcher did not seem to understand the need for a childcare policy to help women carry on with their careers. However, as an older woman, she was stylish and confident. Some would say over-confident or arrogant but this is not meant to be a party political book. So let me just point out that as a menopausal politician, you would never have known that she was in any way menopausal. Yet she must have been at some point during her 'reign'. I suppose then the one thing she may have done for female politicians, is that no one could ever again suggest that older women would be too weak and frail to be at the top of the political world. And she should have opened the door for more female prime ministers. At least we know it's possible now.

WHAT ABOUT OLDER FEMALE POLITICIANS?

We need to encourage women of all ages to go into politics at all levels. Young women who go into politics now will grow older and wiser in the political arena and we will benefit from their experience in the house and as constituent MPs. There are however, a number of older women who enter politics later in life. Back in 2005, Anne Milton became the MP for Guildford aged 55. She later said that people should wait until they were 45 and 'know stuff' before going into politics. She had been a nurse for twenty five years and brought with her a wealth of experience in health and in life. Sheila Gilmore, MP, worked for twenty years in law before going into politics in 2010 and there are many more like her.

You would be forgiven for being unaware of the number of older women entering politics because, surprise surprise, all the publicity tends to go on the younger female new MPs and they are even called 'girls' in the media. Oh joy. And yet, surely, we should be celebrating the women who bring life's experience with them to the political arena.

There are some formidable women politicians who started young but are now in higher positions with a pile of political experience behind them. At the risk of being accused of having some sort of girly crush, Harriet Harman comes to mind. She became an MP back in 1992 and now has that air of experienced and knowledgeable authority we want from our politicians. And as for Shirley Williams, I bow at her feet. She again, has that measured way of talking which comes with age and experience.

We need to be celebrating older women in politics and positions of power. Why is the focus always on the younger females who are still cutting their teeth? We need to value the women who have bought up children, juggled home and work and who have had experience in other work. They have a wide perspective on the world and so have a lot to bring when it comes to making those big decisions.

It used to be that women had more comments made about their appearance than they did on their politics. Even Thatcher was as known for her handbags as her political speeches. I remember jokes about Shirley Williams' hair which seemed to over shadow her politics. And Harriet Harman's shrill voice and Jacqui Smith's low top and so on and so on and so on. Men just never get that sort of press. It seems though that the tide is beginning to change and perhaps we are now listening to women and not just looking at them. This is what I call THE ANGELA MERKEL FACTOR.

No one seems to focus in on what Angela Merkel is wearing or what sort of handbag, if any, she is carrying. We know her as a strong politician and it could be argued Thatcher was also known as a strong politician and yet the focus before Merkel was all about image when it came to the women in positions of power. Merkel represents a shift away from this. I hope. Of course we know, almost unconsciously, that she mostly wears trousers with a selection of jackets and has short hair but without doing a quick internet picture search, I can't for the life of me think if she carries any sort of handbag or what colours she favours. And I most certainly can't recall reading about her appearance or image. I just think of her as confident and smiling and not looking out of place in all those pictures of her with a group of largely male European leaders, while very obviously being a woman.

This is all good news and no one seems sure why this has happened. One thing I have noticed is that comments spread so that once one newspaper hack makes a comment about a politician's appearance, whether it was Shirley Williams' hair or Teresa May's shoes or Jacqui Smith's top, others follow suit. It's lazy journalism and lazy so-called comedy to pick up on one person's comment and just repeat it in an exaggerated form. In other fields, it became trendy to talk about the Duchess of York's very slight weight gain at one point, or suggesting James Blunt can't sing (I've seen him live and boy can he sing) and no one seems to think for themselves any more. Commentators need to comment not just repeat the comments of others. And they need to comment about what's important.

At the time of writing, forty year old Gloria De Piero has just become the new shadow minister for women and equalities. Hooray. I like her. I think she has a chance of doing a good job in that role. But what did one newspaper choose to focus on – the fact that she has chosen not to have children. What has that got to do with her political achievements and abilities? When did you read an article about a male politician who doesn't have children? What a woman chooses to do with her ovaries is private and not really the most important aspect of her promotion. You might as well write about why she doesn't have any pet gerbils, or why she has chosen not to provide shelter for injured Kangaroos in her garage. And other papers have declared they are seeking the topless photos she had taken as a fifteen year old. No, we don't think they're relevant and what she chose to do at fifteen, however misguided (she was fifteen, for goodness sake!) has no bearing on the sort of politician she may be.

Yet I had to check to see if Angela Merkel has children. She doesn't and no one seems that bothered about it. And no doubt she made some dubious choices of one sort or another at fifteen. Didn't we all? So we can only hope that the Angela Merkel way of looking at female politicians continues to spread. I am quietly optimistic but we need to keep a handle on it. Progress can be made and is being made but we can go backwards if we take our eye off the ball.

IN PRAISE OF OLDER WOMEN IN POSITIONS OF POWER

So, like me you sit at home and think of some older woman who's been successful and you might think that you would like to be like her or you might just sit there admiring her. To yourself. And it may be that you've been unaware of a successful woman, whether in politics or in some other field such as science, the arts or business. But then you read about her, or hear a snippet on the radio and then you admire that woman you've just discovered. On your own. To yourself. Well, that's a start and if you're an older, middle-aged woman then that might help you feel good about yourself. It shows older women can get there. Older women can be revered. And you have yourself a role model and you might even feel a little boost of self confidence because of her story. But now you need to SPREAD THE WORD.

We need to be cheerleaders for older women. I don't mean literally. I'm not suggesting you roll up to a local football match waving pom-pom things around shouting 'Two four six eight, who do we appreciate? Germaine Greer.' Or 'give us a C, give us an A…' until you wish you'd chosen someone with a shorter name than Caroline Criado-Perez. I mean we need to tell others about the achievements of older women – maybe those in the political world that you admire or from other walks of life. Maybe even on a very local level by singing the praises of someone who's done well in your town or the company you work for. Tell people you know, put it on social media or start a blog about it. Or write about someone on Wikipedia.

According to the Wall Street Journal, 87% of Wikipedia contributors are male. That's HUGE. And there seems to be a male bias in its content as well, maybe as a result of the overwhelmingly male contributors. The website itself is doing its best to redress this balance with the wikiwomen's collaborative and some publicity from women's groups here and in the USA. It's not clear why there are so few females contributing with many just saying they don't have time. It could be that lack of confidence that still hovers under the surface of so many women – fear of making a mistake and fear of confrontation, which does occur in the arguments on line concerning Wikipedia content. It could also be an awareness of some possible misogynist comments on Wikipedia such as rape scenes in films sometimes being described as sex scenes. But whatever the reason, let's plunge in and change the male bias. It's up to us.

LET'S ALL GET POLITICAL

You may be directly involved in politics in a party political way or you may be a real high flying woman – top of your field. If so, thanks for reading this book. I'm humbled and would like to have coffee some time, talk all this stuff through. For the rest of us, we may think we're on the sidelines. We may admire women in politics (or other high achieving women) and we may support them in whatever way we can but is that enough? There are still older women out there who tell me they're not really political and then go on to tell me they have feminist views. Hang on, if you're a feminist then you are political. Being a feminist is a political statement in that feminists believe in equality for women across the world. There are still some strangely misguided people who don't believe in equality but I can't imagine they are reading this book right now. So if you are a feminist and if you are against ageism then welcome to the world of politics. You don't have to be an MP and you don't even have to support a particular political party to be political. YOU JUST NEED TO WANT TO MAKE THE WORLD A BETTER PLACE. For everyone. And definitely for older women.

Political apathy irritates me. Sorry, but if you are a citizen of this society, the least you can do is care about what's going on around us and how people are treated. The following irritate me so much I find myself screaming at the television. It may have been something I overheard on the bus, but I still scream at the television – it's less confrontational than screaming at a complete stranger. However, if introduced to someone who expresses political apathy, I may scream in their face. Or impose my three hour speech about the matter on them. For your benefit, I have condensed my speech into a handy list of political apatheticals who annoy me:

1. Women who don't vote: Now come on, someone threw themselves under a horse for you. And all you have to do in return is put a cross on a piece of paper.

2. Women who say all politicians are the same: This is far too simplistic. Yes, the parties are all fighting for the middle ground so I take the point, but you need to vote for an MP to represent you. So find out what they might do for you and your town. And if you really can't choose, just go along and spoil your ballot paper. That's a statement in itself and

195

distinguishes you from the 'can't be arsed' brigade.

3. Women who believe we've got there as far as feminism is concerned. The equality laws are in place so why do we still need feminism? Where do I start? While there is FGM, while two women a week are being killed by their partner or ex partner and that doesn't even make the local news, while there are not enough women in Parliament or in board rooms and while it's socially acceptable to stare at pictures of naked breasts while standing at the school gates, we still need it.

4. Women who believe that there is no ageism because we have the law on our side. Sorry, older women in particular are written off too soon, especially in the media and on stage/television.

5. Women who think AA Gill is right about Mary Beard.

6. Older women who think feminism is for younger women. Why? Older women who think they did their bit in the seventies and it's time to let go. Why?

7. Older women, well all women really, in fact everybody and maybe even your pet dog, who live in their own bubble. They might say that violence against women doesn't affect them, they say that they are being treated very well as an older woman in their particular workplace. Or they say life is good here and what are Middle Eastern countries to do with them. DO WE WANT TO LIVE IN A WORLD WHERE THINGS EXIST THAT DEHUMANISE WOMEN? DO WE WANT TO LIVE IN A SOCIETY WHERE THERE IS ANY SORT OF MISOGYNY OR AGEISM OR AGGRESSION TOWARDS WOMEN? Obviously not. Only toddlers are allowed to be 'me, me me' about life. We are grown women. Help make the world a better place or at least care about it. It's what makes us human.

8. Women who are all talk and no action. Now we can't all put

hours of our lives into campaigning on the front line. But if you spend time ranting by the water cooler about some issue or other, then at least put your name on a petition, support women who are out there protesting and campaigning and ask yourself if there's anything, however small, you can do for your cause, which will make the world, the country or just your street a better place. A lot of little actions can make one big action.

9. Women who rant about feminism and ageism and don't walk the walk. Want to change a looks based society? Then why have you booked a Botox appointment?

10. Women who are so wrapped up in their own world, they have to have ten items on a list, even if they can't think of anything different to say for number ten.

POLITICIANS' WIVES AND HUSBANDS

I nearly put politicians' wives under the list of annoying people but then I'm not sure if it's them that annoy me or if it's how the press portray them and I think the latter has more truth about it. As for politicians' husbands, I have to confess I have given them very little thought since Denis Thatcher, so let's start with him.

Whatever your politics, I think many of you will have a bit of a soft spot for good old Denis. He was a real English, slightly eccentric character. And what is more, he was his own man. Happy to stand by Maggie's side, I don't remember him doing that cringey over the top kiss current politicians' wives seem so keen on whenever the cameras are pointing their way. He really seemed to be, well, himself. Supporting Maggie but with no fake gushing shows of solidarity such as staring inanely and adoringly into her eyes. We know he was supportive from what she herself has said and written about him but to be frank, he often looked as if he wished he was at a bar somewhere. Or playing golf. And sometimes that's exactly where he was. The only more current political husband that comes to mind is Jacqui Smith's husband who used tax payers' money to order himself a bit of soft porn to watch. Mostly, we have little interest in the husbands of our more successful female politicians.

To be honest, I don't have all that much interest in political wives either. But the media seem to think we do. And instead of imagining we are interested in their own careers such as Miriam Clegg (also known as Miriam Gonzalez Durantez) being a partner in an international legal practice or Sarah Brown, wife of Gordon Brown, and her charity work and career as a partner in a PR firm, we are told about what they like to wear. In detail.

There are more pictures of Samantha Cameron with headlines entirely concerned with what she's wearing than I care to remember. And naturally, in some of the pictures she is staring adoringly into David's eyes. I wouldn't really mind if they were caught off guard, sharing an intimate loving look as that would seem genuine and rather sweet, but this is posing for the camera to say 'look at us, we're an ordinary couple and not only is David adored as a politician but he still has sex. What more do you want in a prime minister?' You never thought about the sex when you looked at Denis, did you?

So politicians' wives are sort of judged as being someone's wife even if they are successful in their own right. And even if that has a sort of inevitability about it, I do wish they wouldn't milk it. It's a bit demeaning. I would love a politician's wife to be missing from the party conference because she was too busy doing other things. Now, that's an ordinary couple.

The other problem I sometimes have with politicians' wives is when they 'stand by their man.' It's not really the standing by their man as such, which in some instances might be regarded as admirable, it's the *way* they stand by their man. There seems to be some unwritten rule that states when a politician goes astray with another woman, his wife will be there at the gate to their property with a couple of Labradors in the background clinging to her erring husband for dear life. Sometimes with a forced smile on her face. Come on, let's have some honesty about this. What woman would want to come out to the cameras? I'd prefer a more honest picture of her by using a long lens pointed at the kitchen window, where we see her slugging down the gin, mascara running down her face, holding the carving knife and trying to remember if Mrs Bobbitt got off with a caution. It's as if women are forced into a role which they didn't bargain for and in a way men are not.

Middle-aged women in particular will have achieved something themselves without having to resort to being someone's wife and someone's mother. They are so much more than this and deserve recognition as people in their own right. Of course couples want to support each other. But not by false photo opportunities where they are being judged on all the wrong things. And as for the women directly involved, it can be argued that they bring something extra or at least different to politics than your average man.

WHAT WOMEN BRING TO POLITICS

Christine Lagarde, lawyer and once France's finance minister, said that men's ego, sex drive and testosterone made them prone to taking personally decisions that have been made, and to a tendency of humiliating people. She claims that women are less ruled by their libido and are therefore able to make cool-headed judgements.

She may have a point about the sexual libido when you think of the sex scandals that have taken place in politics over the years. From Profumo to Clinton and everyone in between, you wonder if men who make such ill advised decisions in their private life are able to make good political decisions. But can women do better? Is there anything about a woman, and an older woman in particular, that might actually make her a better politician than a man?

There is an argument that women are naturally more caring and nurturing and are more likely to consider the impact of decisions on individuals. Some say a woman could never have done what Blair did in Iraq but then Margaret Thatcher was quite happy to go to war in the Falklands so the argument doesn't really bear out. The only factual differences, as far as the brain is concerned, is that women's language centres are stronger and that men's visual spacial centres are stronger. So men are more likely to be able to read a map and women are more able to talk about the journey. And as being a good orator is part of being a politician, this might give women some advantage when it comes to persuasive speeches.

Margaret Thatcher always banged on about being good at finances because she had to manage the housekeeping. This might be true but I rather wish she hadn't said it. It seemed to label all female politicians as ex housewives for years, which was not all that helpful in the fight for equality.

To be honest, I don't know whether women have extra qualities for the job, I only know that women bring something important to politics – they represent women. Women who have had children and juggled work and home should surely be there helping to make policies about child care, maternity leave and part time working. BUT ALONGSIDE MEN. We need both. As Nancy Astor once said – I can conceive of nothing worse than a man-governed world, except a woman-governed world.

I do though strongly believe that older women have a very important part to play in politics. Their life experience together with a gentle but firm approach to politics has been seen in the likes of Shirley Williams of whom I am something of a fan. And she has the gift of very articulate language which she uses to good effect too.

In October 2013, Time magazine in the USA had the headline – Women are the only adults left in Washington. This followed the sixteen days when America was, well, shut. There were 700,000 workers who had no work or pay for this time. The democrats and republicans couldn't agree a budget plan (all hingeing on Obama's push for a decent health care policy). And guess who came to the rescue? - SuperOlderWoman in the guise of 60 year old Senator from Maine, Susan Collins. She kicked the whole thing off by standing up in the senate and declared that they had to take action to break the deadline. Then a cross party group of FEMALE senators was formed and they worked out a compromise deal. In fact there's a group of women senators known as the sisterhood, who also get together to work out compromises and they have an agreement not to slag each other off in public, despite having differing political views. Sounds good to me. Democrat, Maria Cantwell, said that if women had been left to sort out the deadlock in the first place, it would have been resolved in hours. So maybe women in America bring good skills of compromise and flexibility to the table. But then there's Sarah Palin.

There are a couple of little facts which might make me lean towards the conclusion that women just might make better politicians than men – research shows that men tell twice as many lies as women (though maybe women were too clever to admit it to researchers) and recent research showed that women doctors made better decisions. That might not seem relevant – surely our politicians are not doing hip replacements on the side, but the qualities the study identified were being meticulous about giving the right drugs and referring on to the right specialists. And politicians make life changing decisions too. I retain my view that we need both men and women in politics. Still, women making the best decisions? I wouldn't be at all surprised. And add a bit of experience onto that and I get the impression older women need to take over.

FOURTEEN: WHAT'S IN A NAME?

A 2012 survey carried out by Siteopia.com asked two thousand women what they didn't want to be called. As neither 'slag' nor 'old bag' appeared on the list, I think they were restricting this to terms of endearment (unless women secretly like being called an 'old bag'). In among the top hates were 'babe', 'baby', baby doll' and 'baby girl.' There seems to be a bit of a theme there and I must say I agree. There should, in any case, be an age limit on the use of the word 'babe'. About eighteen months. The other terms women didn't like were all largely sugary food based - such as 'honeybun' or 'sweetie'. Yuk. Although if I'm honest, I don't really like any terms of endearment. So if you meet me, just call me Clare. Not 'honeybun'. And definitely not 'treacle', which was also on the list!

Then there are the casual terms used by people in shops. 'Dear', 'dearie', 'darling' and 'love' are the most used. I have noticed that as I've got older, these terms are used more and more and I really don't like it. I'm not sure if they're ageist terms as such but they might well be. I am sure they are directed more at older women and not so much to younger women or to men of any age but that's just my perception. I'm not sure whether to whinge about this or not as I don't really want to be called 'madam' in shops or restaurants either. How come it sounds so much better in France – 'Madame' in French sounds almost sexy and carries some respect with it, without being patronising. 'Dearie' just doesn't do it. The other thing is how 'love' sounds so much better if you are up North and you can even be called 'pet' without flinching. 'Pet' and 'Love' in Dorking just don't sound right. So are any of these terms ageist or even sexist? I'm not sure they are unless said in a very patronising tone of course. AND

DOES IT MATTER IN THE BIGGER PICTURE OF THINGS?

It seems that we have more important things to worry about. So ignore the man or woman in the bakers who calls you 'my love' (unless he is your love of course). And if it's someone at work you deal with fairly regularly, then just tell them you like being called by your name. Unless you have an embarrassingly awful name in which case I suggest you take any term of endearment you can.

These so called terms of endearment are meant to be just that – endearing. Even if they make you cringe. But there are other terms which fall outside of that category. Rarely said to your face and usually concerned with older women, these are terms such as old bag and old boot or even granny. They are not acceptable and if overheard you may want to say something, particularly if it comes from the mouth of someone you suspect is being judgemental or discriminatory about older people or women or indeed older women. They can be used jokily, I suppose. If I'm in the mood for it.

When it comes to specific labels, women want to be called women according to my own quick survey among anyone who would listen to me. (I asked women obviously, and mainly older women.) Not in 'hey, woman' but as the best choice between that and lady, female or girl. Everyone seems to agree that calling a woman a 'girl' unless she was under sixteen was mostly inappropriate but there seemed to be one exception. Nearly everyone I spoke to admitted that they referred to an all female night out as a 'night out with the girls.' There was some consensus about the word lady. Everyone agreed that they associated the word with a smarmy sort of man who approaches a group of women and says 'hello ladies' in that Leslie Phillips voice. Personally I find it sounds dated and associate it with the phrase 'old lady', for some reason. So women it is. We are women from our late teens until, well, death.

However, there is some confusion when it comes to older women. What do we mean by older? Or middle-aged, for that matter. And do we all mean the same thing? In a recent job I did for the health service I was obliged to attend a number of very dull training days. One of them was called dignity at work. In between naps, I started to listen to the instructions about treating older workers with dignity. And the rule was that you could call someone older but not old. There. Hope that helps in some small way. No, I don't really see the difference either.

What about the term 'middle-aged' and when is it all right to use it? I use it myself and it seems to sum up a group of people in their middle years quite nicely. I am aware that it can be derogatory but this is entirely dependent on the context in which it is being used. 'God, you are so middle-aged' may not be a factual description. It is probably a daughter talking to a mother who hasn't heard of the latest music icon or is wearing the baggy grey cardigan to parents' evening. But 'this book is aimed at middle-aged women' seems pretty factual. Although now I'm thinking I should say 'women in their middle years'. That sounds so much better. Or mid-life woman. No, that sounds like she's half way through her sentence for running over her husband. A woman in her prime is often used to describe a woman who is clearly past her prime, and woman of a certain age means no one knows how old she is and don't want to risk a guess. So let's reclaim the term middle-aged and celebrate those years. When we are a certain age. In our prime. Mid-life.

The trouble is – when exactly is middle-aged? If we knew the date of our death, we could work it out exactly with the use of a decent education or a calculator. But we don't know, so middle-aged is necessarily a band of years. But when does it start and when does it end? That's a bit of a grey area, if you'll pardon the pun.

Research by Age UK, found that more than 45% of 60-64

year olds labelled themselves as middle-aged rather than later life or old age. And I think I would agree with them – being in your sixties certainly isn't later life and definitely not old age. I recall forty being considered middle-aged and if we live till eighty, I suppose there is some accuracy in that. But our life expectancy is going up and forty, in any case, just doesn't have the feel of being middle-aged. With women settling down with a partner at forty or having their first child at forty, as well as going out clubbing and throwing themselves out of aeroplanes and other such stunts, there seems too much that is youthful at forty to use the middle-aged term. So I think middle-aged has shifted up to at least forty-five, maybe later. OK, time to make a decision. I'm going to declare that our middle years (yes, I've decided I prefer that term) start at forty seven. Sounds about right to me

I suppose after our middle years (it's sticking) come our later years, formally known as old age. Obviously, there's no set time for one merging into the other but it certainly isn't in our sixties. Seventy? I'm going to plump for seventy three. So our middle years are roughly from forty seven until seventy three. Approximately. Proving perhaps that terms such as middle-aged (it's back again) and old age are not as useful as we think they are. So best to keep them vague and moveable, I think. Anyway, middle-aged means so much more than an age range. Quite simply, some people are more middle-aged than others. You know the type.

On the whole, I think it's best to use your actual age. This doesn't need to be precise – there is something slightly strange about saying 'I'm fifty six and three quarters' – I find saying that I'm in my fifties is clear enough. I'm not avoiding my precise age but saying things like 'speaking as a woman in her fifties' seems to be enough to make my point. And if my age is irrelevant, then why mention it?

The idea of women keeping their age a secret seems

strange and old fashioned. As if there's some shame in being in your middle or later years. In recent times, I have noticed that people never ask directly 'how old are you?' but 'do you mind telling me your age?', again as if it's a shameful secret. Sometimes, they say it in a whisper as if you are about to disclose something dodgy from your past – a murder perhaps, not the fact that you happened to be born on a certain date.

Having said all that, I have lied about my age. Not because I'm ashamed of it – I mean I've got this far and the alternative isn't a great option. But because I know others will make a judgement about me. As someone who writes plays as well as books, I am aware there has been a big surge towards young playwrights. There are schemes and funding specifically aimed at new playwrights, except that they don't mean new playwrights, they mean young playwrights. So I have lied to enable me to be judged by my work and not my age. But that doesn't really do much good for other older writers coming up behind. So I am slightly embarrassed about lying about my age. However, in cases where age is irrelevant, there is no need to declare it at all. There are so many forms where you are expected to put your age or date of birth. And unless it's for something like a passport or pension scheme, then it's worth taking a moment to decide whether to fill that part of the form in or not. YOU DON'T HAVE TO. This is NOT because you are ashamed of your age, this is because IT'S IRRELEVANT.

So, we are in our middle years, we are not known as dearie or sweetie and we are older rather than old. But most of all we are what we were named at birth. All right, a few of you might have disposed of your birth name in favour of another. I'm thinking of my mother here who was christened Dessica. No, not Jessica which did not come up as a spelling error as I typed it, but Dessica which has come up underlined in red and with a pop up warning, saying 'THIS IS NOT A PROPER NAME'. So she used her middle name, Joyce. Not a great improvement but at least people didn't think she was called Jessica but had a speech problem. And, as the more astute among you will have worked out, I am called Clare and rather more than I am called older or dearie. Except in Asda where dear seems to be the norm. Does my name say anything about me?

In fact names do have a lot to say for themselves. Clare ages me a little as it is less popular among children and there are many Clares of about my age. There are even more Sues. And Debbies. As names go in fashions, people can tell something about your age by your name. So my mother's preferred name of Joyce, firmly placed her in the generation above me, just as there are hardly any Kylies pre-dating Neighbours. There are class issues here too and I'll leave you to debate Camilla versus Cherise and Arabella versus Brittney.

CLICHÉS AND STEREOTYPES

The problem with the label 'middle-aged woman' is that it implies a sort of stereotype, a typical middle-aged woman that describes a whole section of society. There is nothing quite so annoying as lumping a whole group of people together and trying to find some common denominator. This is how we end up with ridiculous, and sometimes dangerous, statements such as 'young people today don't care about politics' or 'Muslims don't like to mix in' or 'Christians are boring.' I have heard all three of those statements on public transport while I have been writing this book, and more. It's a popular pass time of the British to lump a whole section of society, or even a whole population of a country, together and make a sweeping generalisation which can't possibly be true. So sorry Daily Mail readers, but no not all people from Liverpool want to nick your car, and not all people on benefits are lazy. These are lies, laughable though they may be.

When we describe women between forty and sixty (or

my new updated definition of 47 to 73) then we are talking about thousands of people from all backgrounds and walks of life. It would be impossible to lump them all together and describe 'the middle-aged.' And yet people do, both unconsciously and consciously. So, they may or may not be heading for retirement, they may or may not be grey with a thicker stomach, they may have sped up or slowed down, they may be at university or starting a new career, they may or may not be parents or grandparents, they may like Ovaltine (me) or prefer drinking shots in a trendy bar. You cannot make a stereotype out of such a diverse range of women. So don't. And tell other people not to as well. The only thing we all have in common is that we fall into a fairly wide age range. And we've learnt how to laugh at ourselves. Now that can be the new stereotype and I like to think it's an accurate one.

Well done to Lorna Warren and Sheffield University for their Look At Me project which attempts to change that stereotypical image of older women. Although the project has finished, the website is still there for anyone interested.

There are clichés about being middle-aged as well and some are more useful or truthful than others. Here are the top ten, because I like a list and a list of ten in particular. So in at number one...

1. Age is just a number.
Yes, technically it's a number but it's a precise number – the number of years you've been on this earth. We celebrate it in a big way in this society. There are remote tribes that don't celebrate birthdays and as a consequence are unsure how old they are in middle-age and beyond. These are often those same societies where they respect their elders. We could ban birthdays but what would we celebrate instead? The anniversary of the day we started school? (That clearly wouldn't work with the whole country partying in September – on the other hand...) It is just a

number in the sense that once you are past the ages when you can do things for the first time (get married, drink, drive a car, shop in British Home Stores) then how old you are doesn't have to be a restriction on anything you do. You're never too old for anything. Nothing. Not parachute jumping, or listening to One Direction or skateboarding down the corridors at work. Age is a number, not a restriction and not a label. Best get up in the morning, pick a number and be that number for the day. Today I am sixteen which allows me to be both sweet and stroppy. Perfect.

2. You're only as old as you feel.

Yes! I like this one. We can be influenced by society's idea of what we should be like at a certain age. So when you turn sixty, you may feel under some sort of contractual agreement with society that you now need to walk a bit slower (and stop suddenly in the middle of the pavement on a busy High Street), forget where you left your glasses (you'll find them in the fridge) and moan about the price of mint imperials. But you really are as old as you feel so if you are in good health and feel pretty much the same as you did when you were twenty five, then you are indeed twenty five.

3. Getting old is not for the faint hearted.

Actually, life is not for the faint hearted. There are different challenges at different ages. If you sometimes wish you could be a teenager again, stop and give that a bit more thought – do you really want all that angst, all those spots and that amount of complete bewilderment. Trying to make a relationship work, having children, managing your own teenagers – all milestones in life can be looked at with fond affection. But don't forget the sleepless nights and the times you packed your bags and then went back because you didn't want your mother to know you'd had a row with the partner she never liked. Getting older also has its challenges but it's no worse or better than any other section of life. Except you are better equipped to deal with anything that is thrown your way. So enjoy.

4. Youth is wasted on the young.

Yes. When we say we wish we could be young again, what we really mean is that we wish we could be young again WITH HINDSIGHT. I could be a brilliant teenager now, having done it once. Most of us look back at old photos and wonder why we thought we were so ugly at the time, when we had those natural youthful looks. We wonder why an earth we worried so much and didn't enjoy the freedom and lack of responsibility just a bit more. But it's not too late to be youthful. You can be youthful at any age you like and what better time when you have (maybe) lost a bit of that responsibility as your children leave home and you have (maybe) paid off the mortgage. So get a pogo stick, take up street dancing, buy a motorbike and go off somewhere, and paint a ceiling black. Anything you like. But don't take on the aspects of youth you don't want. No need to be painfully awkward in order to re-capture that youthful feeling.

5. Older and Wiser.

Usually. We've all met people who make the same mistakes over and over again and don't seem to learn from them. I know someone who has gone through life marrying the same man. I don't mean literally – she didn't keep marrying Kenny every year because she had a penchant for wedding cake, white clothes and family arguments, but she married the same type. They even looked like Kenny. But more importantly, they were men who liked to control her and were very jealous and I mean VERY jealous. She can not live with a man who needs to know where she is every second of the day and who could? But yet she married the same jealous type over and over. Well, three times anyway. So not older and wiser then. Experience should make us wiser but only if WE LEARN FROM OUR MISTAKES. We all have instances when we haven't learnt lessons from our errors, it's as if life throws us the same challenge again and again until we finally get it. We diet, we err, diet again. You know Scotch makes you feel ill but someone offers you a twenty five year old single malt and you know this time will be different. But no, you feel sick again. (All right, that one's about me). You know you don't feel comfortable in a polo neck as it makes your neck itch but you buy another one because you like the colour (me, again). You know eating cheese make you snore and makes you hot but you have a pile of cheese and biscuits before going to bed anyway (not me, but someone I know rather well). If you keep doing the same thing, you will get the same result. So to be older and wiser, make some changes, use the experience you have accumulated for your own good and for the greater good.

6. Good things come to those who wait.

Maybe. But maybe 'good things come to those who persevere' would be a better saying. If you sit around waiting, nothing much will happen. But if that waiting includes a bit of action then yes, you will get there. We have already discussed older women who achieved success in their field later in life – this didn't come about by just waiting around long enough, it came about because of perseverance and hard work. And patience. And never giving up. Buses come to those who wait long enough. Cold feet will come to those who wait around in the cold. Long hair and long nails come to those who wait. But everything else requires a bit of effort. I also think that believing it will come will help enormously.

7. The only certainty is death.

The main certainty is death. The others are 1) you will get older 2) you will drive or walk past a Tescos more frequently than you will be aware of 3) you will know the end to every Hollywood Rom Com within five minutes of starting to watch it 4) you will have at least one TV programme you secretly watch but slag off to all your friends 5) there will be occasions when you can't be done with the recycling and shove it all in one black bag. But death is the main one.

8. Growing old is mandatory, growing up is optional.

I like this one. It's sort of true. You can act any way you want. But you won't get to your middle years without a few traumas and challenges along the way. Show me an older woman who has not had at least one major struggle or knock back in her life and I will show you a liar. And these events tend to make us grow up a lot. But get in touch with your inner child on a daily basis. But don't call it an inner child if you are British – think of something else to call it. Your fun soul, perhaps.

9. Old enough to know better.

You will carry on making mistakes for your entire life. That's life – you wake up, make a few mistakes, have your tea and go to bed. Every day. But you will slowly learn from your mistakes, and you WILL get better at covering up your blunders.

10. Middle-age is when your age starts to show around your middle.

This is a Bob Hope quote and no book should be complete without one. It also gives me a chance to share an interesting fact with you. Waists in middle-aged women are getting larger and have grown by quite a bit since the 1950s (the average size has apparently gone up by six inches since then). This isn't really very surprising – everyone's waists are getting bigger so why should we be an exception?

We have looked at middle-age and decided you might or might not want to call it something else. But the next question has to be – when do we drift into old age? I have suggested seventy three and yet I know some very sprightly seventy three year olds. I suppose old age comes when you start to become a bit more dependent on others. I have to admit I haven't given my old age any thought at all. Except to deny it will happen, much as we tend to deny death will happen. But I have to think about it now as I have decided it needs its own chapter.

FIFTEEN: GETTING EVEN OLDER

My own parents had short illnesses and both died in their early eighties, very neatly and conveniently (in some ways) a matter of weeks apart. They only became dependent on myself and my brothers for a matter of about three or four months. It seemed never ending at the time – starting with driving them to endless medical appointments and finishing up with me staying most nights there to look after my father while my mother was, unknown to us, quietly dying herself. But it was, in comparison with others, a very short period of dependence. When my father died, I imagined I would be spending every weekend sorting my mother out as my father had dealt with pretty much everything. He even had to show her how to put petrol in the car when he knew he had limited life. She was particularly hopeless at anything to do with bills and money. I am sure it was my husband John telling my mother that he was setting her up on digital banking which finally finished her off.

Before those few months of illness and dying, my parents were not old. They were both driving round, they went away for weekends, they were only very slightly forgetful and were enjoying life. Others of exactly the same age are already old and dependent. It seems old age comes at different times for different people (a bit like middle-age). So we can only hope to delay the dependent brand of old age for as long as possible. Some of this might be influenced by our genes, but there are also things we can do to keep that dependent old age at bay. And it starts in mid life.

While I strongly advocate living in the present moment, even living each day as if it might be your last, it probably won't be your last. So it doesn't seem incongruent to keep one eye on the future. That's why we should have all written our wills, left any instructions for our deaths and funerals and made any decisions about what we want when we become more dependent. For some this might mean a living will. We can also take steps to ensure we have the best chance of living independently as long as possible.

1. Keep fit NOW. Make walking, cycling, netball, extreme ironing up mountains, jumping up and down on the car, or whatever your fitness choice is, part of your life. So much easier to continue with this when our bones get a bit creaky than to suddenly take it up. And remember, you won't keep up with anything you hate. So find something that you enjoy. If the word fitness makes you reach for a doughnut and a glass of red, then work out how you will make yourself indulge in a bit of movement – dancing? Running up stairs? If you hate it all, then do it right before your favourite TV programme so that you have something to look forward to and don't allow yourself to watch it unless you've jogged around a bit first. Delayed gratification – works a treat.

2. Use it or lose it. For the mind as well as the body. Read, learn, go to classes, travel, do something new.

3. Change your routine from time to time. Even small things like taking a different route to the shops, changing your supermarket, moving the furniture around or standing on your head to clean your teeth. Change keeps us alert.

4. Work out in advance how you want to spend your time when you're retired. Lying on a sun lounger drinking Pina Coladas is not a realistic option. Especially if you retire in February. And you live in Aberdeen. Seriously, you will get bored, unfit and mentally stale. And if you don't make some sort of plan, you will suddenly find a big hole in your life. Many women get depressed when they retire. They've relished the idea for months, even years, and then it doesn't live up to any sort of expectation. So take up something new as well as sort out the

loft. Extend your hobby or take up a new one, do some voluntary work – it really won't feel like actual work because you're THERE BY CHOICE.

5. Think ahead to when you are slightly slower and a little bit older. No need to get the stair lift fitted and a hoist to get yourself out of bed if you don't need them because you might NEVER need them. My parents spent the last five years of their life obsessed with what would happen when they couldn't make it up the stairs. Their stairs wouldn't really take a stair lift so they started looking for a bungalow to buy. But they never needed a stair lift. Their legs were their greatest assets. It was other parts of them which were falling apart. However, you might want to think hard if you live miles from any facilities or other people. There is a danger of getting isolated or reliant on the car. Other than that, if you like where you live, stay there. But if you'd lived there purely because of your work or good local schools, think about a change. And in making your change, visualise yourself living there in ten, twenty and thirty years' time.

6. For most people, the aim is to stay living in your own home until the end, or at least for as long as possible. So make sure your home is suitable for you as you get older – don't be coy about getting hand rails and the like fitted to make life easier later. You can think about which care home you'd like but just jot some thoughts down on a piece of paper for now and put it in a drawer or give it to a younger family member. Don't dwell on it as you may never need to make that choice. That's plan B, and plan A is the aim.

7. We aren't all going to make it to the end physically and mentally intact. You can register with the Public Guardian to allow someone to make choices for you should you lose your mental capacity. Like making a will, or funeral preparations – do it, just in case.

8. Accept help. Sounds simple but many women get more stubborn as they get older. It pained my mother to ask me for help even if it was just a lift to an appointment. She never liked to bother me and would talk about taxis and the like. Why? I was more than happy to step in. It's something about reversing the roles. I had a bit of a taste for that following an operation to remove a tumour in my leg. My daughters rallied round and my youngest daughter was at home doing the cooking and ironing for me. At first IT FELT SO WRONG. I should have been looking after her – that's what mothers do. Even though she was in her twenties so hardly a child carer. Yet, she has told me that she enjoyed 'looking after me'. And has volunteered to look after me when I'm old, should I need it. (I must remember to get that in writing.) So take help from family, friends and neighbours. You will soon sense if you are asking too much.

9. Practice being eccentric and, if you choose, cantankerous. Old age is when you can say what you like and people will laugh. Like childhood but with worse teeth. Have you always wanted to tell your neighbour he's the dullest man on earth and his car won't explode if he doesn't polish it three times a week? Then wait until you're old enough. That's what I'm doing. And wear a ridiculous hat. Why? Because you can.

10. Make sure you are set up with technology. You will need the internet even more when you are older. And a phone you can have right next to you. Maybe an iPad. Whatever you can afford to have. And keep up with the latest – there'll be more changes before you reach old age, so if they invent a mobility scooter that shouts out abuse as you speed along, or an iron you can work from a remote control while you sit in front of the telly or a wrist watch that re-writes your will every time a family member annoys you, then save up for it.

There was a TV programme not so long ago where old people from a care home were put in a house together to, well, fend for themselves. The results were amazing. Much to their surprise, they soon found themselves cooking and flying up stairs they had thought they couldn't manage and more importantly, they became more mentally alert. Because they had to be. Just saying. Just warning.

THAT DIFFICULT CONVERSATION
There is a Danish saying which roughly translates as 'Make your decisions before others make them for you.' A recent survey by Anchor (a not for profit housing organisation) found that two thirds of us have not had a proper conversation about what we want in old age. Presumably those questioned were approaching old age, not fourteen year olds who might legitimately have more pressing concerns. For the middle-aged women among you, this might be the conversation you have with your parents. And later, it will be the conversation you have with your offspring or younger friends and relatives. You make provision for your pension as soon as you start work, so why not for your care and ultimately death.

1. Have that conversation and make sure it concerns practicalities.
2. The longer you leave it, the harder the conversation will be and the more rushed it will seem.
3. There are plenty of options from staying in your own home with support to care homes to rented sheltered accommodation.
4. Plenty of funeral options too - consider them all.
5. Think about a living will in case you end up very ill and not wanting to carry on.
6. Write a will, whatever your age. No reason not to.

7. Avoiding thinking about death? Admit it and make yourself confront it. After all, it's an inevitability not a possibility.
8. As you get older, think about the all important details. There was a picture in the press recently of a dying elderly woman in a hospital bed who had been taken outside (in the bed) to say goodbye to her horse. Good on the hospital and good on the woman for knowing this was what she needed.

FEMINISM AND THE ELDERLY

It's a sad fact of life that elderly women are still at risk of rape. The home office has no figures as rape crimes are not categorised by age. However, judging by press reports, this is a growing problem. Unlike rapes in younger women, there has been no real research into this area. We don't talk about it much while other sorts of rape are under a lot of discussion. It's back to not wanting to associate older people with the sexual act, even though it's really violence we're talking about. And it's about people not understanding why a young man would even WANT to rape an old woman. With no research, we can only speculate that it might be the vulnerability of an older woman (rape being as much about power as sex) or that the rapist might have a problem with older people who represent authority. It has a different profile than other rapes. Usually, in fact between sixty and seventy percent of cases, the rape victim knows the rapist. But in the elderly, it tends to be a break in by a stranger.

Is this a feminist or an ageist issue? Both. Women, particularly older women living on their own, have the right to feel safe in their own homes, or walking down the street for that matter. And we need to look after our elderly in this society. Surely some research needs to be carried out to find what makes a young man rape an elderly woman? Knowledge and understanding is the first step towards any kind of attempt to change behaviours and cultures, and knowledge of why a man might rape an older woman might be particularly relevant in our understanding of rape as power and violence rather than sexual. It might help us to move away from the 'she was asking for it' culture or even, the 'all men are rapists' idea. So why the lack of research or even interest in what seems to be a growing problem? This is most certainly a feminist issue.

The elderly are feminists too. It doesn't just stop when you get to a certain age. And if you are a feminist, and I imagine you are, then you still will be however old you grow. Even if we have reached total equality (ha ha) then we still need to maintain that equality. And it's essential that any feminist movement is all inclusive – all backgrounds, all cultures, all religions, ALL AGES. All the issues that concern younger feminists still concern older feminists and there are some issues specifically about the elderly to consider.

One of the main issues is who looks after you as you get older. Because, the chances are very high that it will be a woman. Traditionally, women have always tended to take on the caring roles, but how is it that so many women also take on the responsibility for their in-laws? When we talk about the sandwich generation, we describe a woman caught between her teenage children and HER ageing parents. But it could just as well be HIS ageing parents. If you have a son, is it really his wife you want doing all the supporting stuff? If you feel guilty about asking your son for help, then at least you can remind yourself of all you did for him as he grew up. Seems to be redressing the balance or something. And you may well imagine resentment from a daughter in law, whether she feels it or not.

If you have sons, it might be a good idea to discuss this well in advance of getting old. Some men are not all that good at seeing what might be needed and will need a very direct conversation. You don't want to wait until you're ninety and your daughter in law has decided to completely rearrange your flat while all you can do is drop hints.

No doubt as well, people will still be focusing on the older women who happen to look young for their age. Swop 'she looks amazing for fifty' for 'she looks amazing for eighty' and you may feel your alert mind is of no importance at all (it is). It won't be long before the red tops are taking photos of some female celebrity in her coffin and writing the headline 'looks amazing for a corpse.'

When you consider people in their eighties and nineties, it could be argued that all issues about care of the elderly are feminist issues, simply because most of the elderly population will be women. We still live, on average, much longer than men and it's more often or not women who have been in a long term (or short term) partnership who will be the ones learning to live alone. So, think ahead and work out how you intend to live as you age. And fight against sexism and ageism until the day you die. Or beyond – you can always ask for some quotes from Germaine Greer or Simone de Beauvoir at your funeral.

SIXTEEN: A MIDDLE-AGED MANIFESTO

WHAT DO WE WANT!

1. Respect for everyone whatever their age or sex (or background, sexuality, ethnicity).
2. A society which values experience.
3. Media which focuses on the achievements of older women, not just pictures of how they look remarkably young for their age.
4. Photo shopped pictures to be labelled in BIG writing that they are photo shopped and therefore not a true likeness to the original.
5. A society which is not horrified by the signs of ageing. Grey hair and wrinkles are natural signs of ageing. No shame. Just choice.
6. Visual media who do not discriminate against older women. Why is it alright to have a grey, slightly lined David Dimbleby on our screens while Mary Beard is berated?
7. A society where everyone mixes in together, whatever their age.
8. Reinforcement and awareness of existing ageism and sexism laws.
9. More portrayal of older women in the arts (theatre, film, TV drama) in a positive light and showing older women as active, sexual and assertive, not just victims or someone's Mum or wife.
10. Older women who feel safe, respected and an integral part of our society.

WHEN DO WE WANT IT?
Now.

HOW DO WE GET IT?

Keep campaigning, increase awareness of successful older women, fight against sexism and ageism both locally, nationally and internationally. And be a good advocate for older women by being who you are and having fun while you're being you.

And now a list of animals. Why not?

1. Be a Butterfly

I don't mean flit about looking for something sweet to nibble on (although that's not a bad way of life). Native Americans say that the butterfly teaches us that change may be painful but is necessary. And if you think about the butterfly – there is beauty in reaching maturity. And we don't compare butterflies and say one is more beautiful than another, or one has obviously let herself go. When I went recently to the butterfly tent at the Natural History Museum, the joy was in the diversity of the butterflies. Caterpillars are really just there getting ready to be butterflies. The symbolism goes on and on. So transform yourself, re-invent yourself and find a new, deeper kind of beauty. But know that you are still the same creature that you always were, just more flamboyant.

2. Be a kangaroo

Kangaroos can't go backwards. OK, they can turn round and walk back the way they came but for all intents and purposes, they can only move forward. And that's a good way to live as a middle-aged and older woman. The only certainty is that things will change (all right, there's death too) and we can not go back to 'how things were'. There is nothing as ageing as someone stuck in the past. Reminisce if you want to, remember if you can, but embrace today and look forward to the future. And keep hopping.

3. Be a chameleon

Keep adapting yourself as you go through the major milestones of children leaving home, retirement and so on. And adapt your environment as well to suit you.

4. Be a chimpanzee

Have fun. Laugh at life. We're surely here to be happy. As women, we often see ourselves as carers – ensuring those around us are happy and content and not focusing on ourselves. Nothing wrong with that, but happiness spreads so you can bring joy to others simply by being joyful yourself, so it is in no way a self-centred state to be in. And if there are people in this world who think older women are moany and whingey, prove them wrong.

5. Be a Dolphin

Many people get the wrong idea about dolphins. They assume they are fish just because they live in the ocean but they are not fish at all. That's the wrong label. You may think they just swim about but they love to play. They are far more intelligent than we often give them credit for and they have a tendency to do surprising things like rescue people from drowning. Older women have a stereotype attached to them – an invisible, insignificant woman who likes to drink Horlicks and watch Emmerdale. Wrong. The wrong label. We have so much to offer so be who you are and do your bit to break down those stereotypes and misconceptions.

6. Be a moth

Some people might think a moth is a moth. Just the one. Sort of brown and insignificant. Hardly notice them, really. But there are 160,000 different species of moths in the world, all different shapes and sizes but united under the one label of moth. Like older women. We are all different, you cannot make generalisations or assumptions about us. So don't let people do it.

7. Be a bee

Keep busy, keep active, keep thinking.

8. Be a howler monkey

Spot an injustice? A blatant bit of sexism and/or ageism? Then don't just moan in the small bar of the Wig and Fidget, SHOUT ABOUT IT. Write to your MP, boss, local feminist group, tweet it and so on. Nothing changes without the will to change it and the action to make sure it gets changed. Remember, nearly all social changes in the world started with protests or rebellions. Change doesn't tend to happen quietly.

9. Be a squirrel

Prepare for the winter of your life. That's almost poetic, so I think I'll leave it there.

10. Be an elephant

There's some great footage of elephants teaching their young how to use their trunks and how to cover themselves in mud to protect themselves from sunburn. You will have acquired an enormous amount of life experience and knowledge over the years so pass it on.

SEVENTEEN: CELEBRATE

We have come a long way. We know that because there was a time when there were no equality laws, women earned significantly less than men for doing EXACTLY the same job and laws around maternity pay and conditions weren't there. At one time, women couldn't vote or inherit or do anything much without the permission of men. So, yes we have come a long way even if some new, very modern causes for concern have emerged in the mean time.

Feminism is described as coming in three waves. First, suffragettes fought hard for equal voting rights, then laws changed in the nineteen sixties to eighties and now we find ourselves on the crest of the third wave. I imagine awareness of inequalities came long before the suffragettes, perhaps with stone age women protesting that the men got to go out hunting while they were tied to the kitchen fire. Then historical events had their impact, the most obvious being the world wars when women got a taste for work, money and independence. Over the course of history, there have no doubt been women as well as men who simply accepted the status quo and had to have the inequalities pointed out to them. Even now, a lot of the campaigning being done is about awareness.

The same goes for older women. We have known for some time that older women tend to become invisible but it's as if each woman has to experience that change for herself before she sits up and realises that something needs to improve. It's largely a matter of changing attitudes and that tends to be a gradual process. And that's what this book is all about – opening up the debate and changing attitudes towards middle-aged and older women. I don't imagine as a result of this book, I will suddenly be respected for my experience and not treated like an idiot in shops. But there will be some shifting as there is already.

This new wave of feminism is trying to be all inclusive and has certainly raised awareness, especially of the more serious issues. While we have teenage girls depressed because they feel judged by their appearance, while we have boys learning about sex from violent porn or porn that demeans women, while we have forced marriages, FGM and countries where women are not even allowed to drive, while we have ongoing domestic violence largely aimed at women and while we have a predominance of men in the boardroom or in parliament, we still need feminism. Feminism to increase awareness, take action and instigate some changes. And while we have older male presenters on TV but very few older women, while older women are portrayed as stereotypes in drama, and while older women are losing confidence and even becoming clinically depressed because of the focus on having youthful looks, then we have an ageism problem on top of this. Middle-aged women and older women feel invisible and so they retreat into their homes even though they have a wealth of experience and knowledge to share with the world. But we are beginning to come out of our shells and start shouting – here we are, we're important and get used to us because there's going to be a whole lot more of us very soon.

Middle-aged and older women are wonderful Why? We need a final list.

1. Older women are funny. They make me laugh. I make people laugh. It seems to be a well kept secret that a group of older women can make each other (and others) laugh till they cry. I think they are funnier than men, they just don't need to tell stupid jokes. They see the funny side of life, are very adept at relaying hilarious anecdotes and can laugh at themselves.
2. Older women are wise. We are good at learning from our mistakes (usually), we accumulate knowledge and experience and adapt to new situations.

3. Older women are aware. We make inequalities of all kinds our business and we want to change things.

4. Older women are angry. We don't want to be invisible. We don't want to be written off. We don't want to STILL be judged on how young for our age we look.

5. Older women look great. Some may look young for their age, most won't, some may choose to dye their hair, others won't. We come in all shapes and sizes but if we are NOT bombarded with criticism and negativity, then we have the ability to BLOSSOM as we get older.

6. Older women can do anything. We are not restricted by age, so don't put restrictions out there for us.

7. Older women have fought before. Many of us were part of the second wave of feminism and so it seems natural to be part of the third wave. Some things have changed, some things have not. We're onto it.

8. Older women like younger women. And men of all ages. We are not a separate species.

9. Older women may have had similar numbers of birthdays, but apart from that we are as diverse as the rest of you. I know a rather dull twenty five year old who can't think for herself. There are people like that in every age group just as there are dynamic, shape shifting, big personalities in every generation.

10. We are the generation who don't have to have their pubic hair removed or shaved into the shape of a small animal.

11. Older women aren't old at all really. Their bodies may have a bit of wear and tear, their minds may or may not need some reminders every now and then. But middle-aged and older women are youthful underneath.

So there we have it, older women are wonderful and we should ensure every one celebrates that fact and embraces us.

Literally. While, of course, keeping our eye on out of date, misguided attitudes that label and hurt us. And to make sure men are included in this debate, we will finish with quotes from three of them.

'You don't stop laughing when you grow old, you grow old when you stop laughing.' George Bernard Shaw
'The afternoon knows what the morning never suspected.' Robert Frost.
'Older women. Of which I count myself one. In front of the telly, I'm transgender and menopausal.' AA Gill. (Sunday Times October 13) Now completely forgiven.

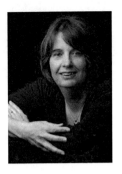

Clare Shaw was born in Cornwall and has been writing for as long as she remembers. Her first books were four Parenting books, published by Hodder which she wrote after a stint working for 'Parents' and 'Practical Parenting' magazines.

In 2008, she had her novel 'The Mother and Daughter Diaries' published and began to write plays, her first was performed at Barnes Arts Centre. Her plays have been performed at venues such as The Pleasance and New Wimbledon studio theatre. Her radio play, 'Selling Shoes in Southend', was produced by Frequency Theatre as a result of being one of the winners in a competition with Essex Books Festival in conjunction with the BBC. A radio play was broadcast on Radio North.

Clare lives in Essex with John and has two daughters.